Emergency Approaches to Neurosurgical Conditions

Abhishek Agrawal • Gavin Britz
Editors

Emergency Approaches to Neurosurgical Conditions

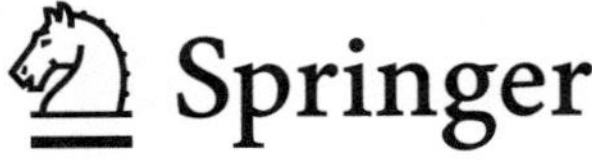 Springer

Editors
Abhishek Agrawal, M.D
Department of Neurosurgery
and Radiology
Brigham and Women's Hospital
Harvard Medical School
Boston, MA
USA

Gavin Britz
Department of Neurosurgery
Methodist Neurological Institute
Houston, TX
USA

ISBN 978-3-319-10692-2   ISBN 978-3-319-10693-9   (eBook)
DOI 10.1007/978-3-319-10693-9
Springer Cham Heidelberg New York Dordrecht London

Library of Congress Control Number: 2014958084

© Springer International Publishing Switzerland 2015
This work is subject to copyright. All rights are reserved by the Publisher, whether the whole or part of the material is concerned, specifically the rights of translation, reprinting, reuse of illustrations, recitation, broadcasting, reproduction on microfilms or in any other physical way, and transmission or information storage and retrieval, electronic adaptation, computer software, or by similar or dissimilar methodology now known or hereafter developed. Exempted from this legal reservation are brief excerpts in connection with reviews or scholarly analysis or material supplied specifically for the purpose of being entered and executed on a computer system, for exclusive use by the purchaser of the work. Duplication of this publication or parts thereof is permitted only under the provisions of the Copyright Law of the Publisher's location, in its current version, and permission for use must always be obtained from Springer. Permissions for use may be obtained through RightsLink at the Copyright Clearance Center. Violations are liable to prosecution under the respective Copyright Law.
The use of general descriptive names, registered names, trademarks, service marks, etc. in this publication does not imply, even in the absence of a specific statement, that such names are exempt from the relevant protective laws and regulations and therefore free for general use.
While the advice and information in this book are believed to be true and accurate at the date of publication, neither the authors nor the editors nor the publisher can accept any legal responsibility for any errors or omissions that may be made. The publisher makes no warranty, express or implied, with respect to the material contained herein.

Printed on acid-free paper

Springer is part of Springer Science+Business Media (www.springer.com)

Preface

Patients with neurosurgical conditions are almost always referred from either primary care physicians, neurologists, internist, or a specialist in family medicine. This two-volume guide will answer commonly asked questions about neurosurgical conditions related to brain and spinal cord, in an attempt to fill in the gap and answer numerous questions that arise after a diagnosis is made, explaining the basics of neurosurgical disease spectrum and their management options.

Comprehensive Guide to Neurosurgical Conditions (*Volume I*) updates the reader on basic neuroanatomy and physiology, including general neurosurgical conditions, ideal neurosurgical and intensive care unit set up, second opinion, brain death, and organ donation in a comprehensive and concise manner.

Comprehensive Guide which is part of a book set including *Emergency Approaches to Neurosurgical Conditions* (*Volume II*) delves into different kinds of complex brain surgeries and focuses on the surgical aspect of neurosurgical conditions, including management of tumors, aneurysms, and pediatric conditions in chapters written by reputed neurosurgeons in their allied subspecialty.

This two-volume book set also aims to replace "excess-information" obtained on the internet about a particular neurosurgical disease, which may be too overwhelming, not complied properly, not updated, or may be misinterpreted, misunderstood, or irrelevant for that particular disease. This concise book is intended not only for neurologists or neurosurgeons who have direct patient interaction but also for brain surgery patients and their families, medical students, paramedics, nurse practitioners, physician assistants, health planners, residents, and fellows who are already trained or in training, to get a quick glimpse of neurosurgical conditions encountered on a day-to-day basis.

Boston, MA, USA   Abhishek Agrawal
Houston, TX, USA   Gavin Britz

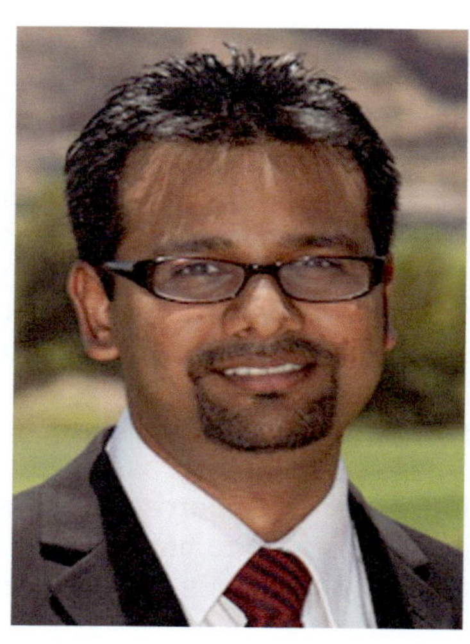

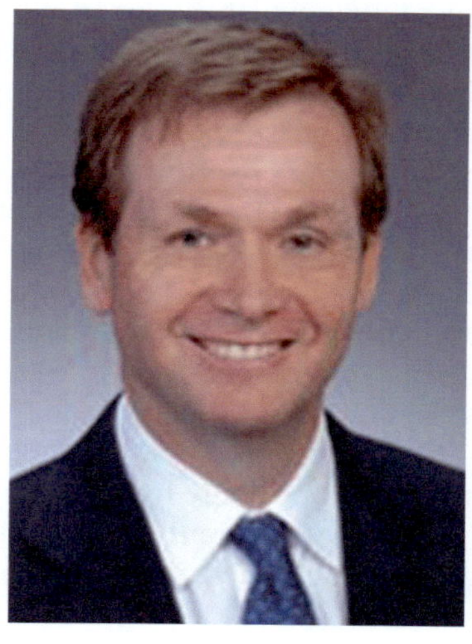

Acknowledgments

The key to success of any project depends upon the inputs and guidance received from persons associated with the project. Fortunately for us, there was encouragement, guidance, and support from all quarters of life.

Great are those who teach and inspire. They deserve gratitude which can be expressed at a time like this. Our inestimable gratitude goes to our colleagues and authors who spend their precious time contributing chapters for this book.

We are also thankful to our assistant, Peggy Kelly, who managed to keep track of the chapters and authors. In addition, we would like to express our gratitude to Melissa Morton, Julia Megginson, and R. Nithyatharani from Springer Publishers for their collegiality.

Behind all this is the unconditional support, motivation, and encouragement from our family members, parents, and children who have always been a source of strength and inspiration.

Abhishek Agrawal
Gavin Britz

Contents

Contributors

Vijay Agarwal, MD Division of Neurological Surgery, Department of Surgery, Duke University Medical Center, Durham, NC, USA

Anthony M. Avellino, MD, MBA Department of Neurological Surgery, University of Washington School of Medicine, Seattle, WA, USA

David S. Baskin, MD Department of Neurosurgery, Houston Methodist Hospital, Houston, TX, USA

Teresa E. Bell-Stephens, RN, BSN, CNRN Department of Neurosurgery, Stanford University School of Medicine, Stanford, CA, USA

Mitchel S. Berger, MD Department of Neurological Surgery, University of California, San Francisco, San Francisco, CA, USA

J. Bob Blacklock, MD Department of Neurosurgery, Methodist Neurological Institute, Houston, TX, USA

Kelly Blessing, FNP Department of Neurology, Duke University Medical Center, 2900 Bryan Research Building Research Drive, Durham, NC, USA

Gavin Britz, MD Department of Neurosurgery, Houston Methodist Hospital, Houston, TX, USA

Imran Chaudry, MD Department of Radiology, Medical University of South Carolina, Charleston, SC, USA

Susan Chioffi, RN, MSN, ACNP-BC Department of Neurology, Duke University Medical Center, Durham, NC, USA

Graham H. Creasey, MB, ChB, FRCSEd Department of Neurosurgery, Stanford University School of Medicine, VA Palo Alto Health Care System, Stanford, Palo Alto, CA, USA

Videndra Desai, MD Department of Neurosurgery, Houston Methodist Hospital, Houston, TX, USA

Virendra Desai, MD Department of Neurosurgery, Methodist Neurological Institute, Houston, TX, USA

Orlando Diaz, MD Department of Neurosurgery, Houston Methodist Hospital, Houston, TX, USA

Richard G. Ellenbogen, MD, FACS Department of Neurological Surgery, University of Washington Medicine, Seattle, WA, USA

Herbert E. Fuchs, MD, PhD, FAANS, FAAP Department of Surgery, Duke Medical Center, Durham, NC, USA

Carmelo Graffagnino, MD Department of Neurology, Duke University Medical Center, 2900 Bryan Research Building Research Drive, Durham, NC, USA

Gerald A. Grant, MD, FACS Department of Neurosurgery, Stanford University Medical Center/Lucile Packard Children' Hospital, Standord, CA, USA

Mary Guhwe, RN, MSN, FNP-BC, SCRN Department of Neurology, Duke University Medical Center, Durham, NC, USA

Mihir Gupta, BA School of Medicine, Stanford University, Palo Alto, CA, USA

Samuel Braydon Harris Columbia University, New York, USA

Shawn L. Hervey-Jumper, MD Department of Neurological Surgery, University of California, San Francisco, San Francisco, CA, USA

Paul J. Holman, MD Department of Neurosurgery, Methodist Neurological Institute, Houston, TX, USA

Daniel S. Ikeda, MD Department of Neurological Surgery, The Ohio State University's Wexner Medical Center, Columbus, OH, USA

Robert E. Isaacs, MD Division of Neurological Surgery, Department of Surgery, Duke University Medical Center, Durham, NC, USA

Richard P. Klucznic, MD Department of Neurosurgery, Houston Methodist Hospital, Houston, TX, USA

Brandon D. Liebelt Department of Neurosurgery, Methodist Neurological Institute, Houston, TX, USA

Evan S. Marlin, MD Department of Neurological Surgery, The Ohio State University's Wexner Medical Center, Columbus, OH, USA

Matthew McLaurin, MD Louisiana State University, Baton Rouge, LA, USA

Ciarán J. Powers, MD Department of Neurological Surgery, The Ohio State University's Wexner Medical Center, Columbus, OH, USA

Leonardo Rangel-Castilla, MD Division of Neurological Surgery, c/o Neuroscience Publications, Barrow Neurological Institute, St. Joseph's Hospital and Medical Center, Phoenix, AZ, USA

Andrew B. Shaw, MD Department of Neurological Surgery, The Ohio State University's Wexner Medical Center, Columbus, OH, USA

Robert F. Spetzler, MD Division of Neurological Surgery, c/o Neuroscience Publications, Barrow Neurological Institute, St. Joseph's Hospital and Medical Center, Phoenix, AZ, USA

Alejandro M. Spiotta, MD Department of Neurosurgery, Medical University of South Carolina, Charleston, SC, USA

Blake Staub, MD Department of Neurosurgery, Methodist Neurological Institute, Houston, TX, USA

Gary K. Steinberg, MD,PhD Department of Neurosurgery, Stanford University School of Medicine, Stanford, CA, USA

Todd S. Trask, MD Department of Neurosurgery, Methodist Neurological Institute, Houston, TX, USA

Aquilla S. Turk, DO Department of Radiology and Radiological Sciences, Medical University of South Carolina, Charleston, SC, USA

Raymond Turner, MD Department of Neurosurgery, Medical University of South Carolina, Charleston, SC, USA

Jan Vargas, MD Department of Radiology and Radiological Sciences, Medical University of South Carolina, Charleston, SC, USA

Alexander West, MD Department of Neurosurgery, Houston Methodist Hospital, Houston, TX, USA

Yi Jonathan Zhang, MD Department of Neurosurgery, Methodist Neurological Institute, Houston, TX, USA

Chapter 1
Non-malignant Brain Tumors

Shawn L. Hervey-Jumper and Mitchel S. Berger

Abbreviations

CT	Computed tomography
DTI	Diffusion tensor imaging
IDH	Isocitrate dehydrogenase
MRI	Magnetic resonance imaging
NF2	Neurofibromatosis type 2
PCV	Procarbazine carmustine and vincristine
SRS	Stereotactic radiosurgery
WHO	World Health Organization

Introduction

Non-malignant tumors of the brain and central nervous system occur at an incidence of 17.9 per 100,000 in the United States [25, 26]. The most common primary non-malignant tumors are gliomas and meningiomas [25, 26]. Gliomas are tumors intrinsic to the brain that arise from glial cells (supporting cells), and include astrocytomas, oligodendroglioma,

S.L. Hervey-Jumper, MD • M.S. Berger, MD (✉)
Department of Neurological Surgery, University of California,
San Francisco, San Francisco, CA, USA
e-mail: bergerm@neurosurg.ucsf.edu

A. Agrawal, G. Britz (eds.), *Emergency Approaches to Neurosurgical Conditions*, DOI 10.1007/978-3-319-10693-9_1,
© Springer International Publishing Switzerland 2015

and mixed tumors (oligoastrocytomas). Meningiomas arise outside of the brain from arachnoidal cells of the meninges (coverings of the brain). They represent the most frequently diagnosed brain tumors in adults, accounting for 28–35 % of cases [25, 26, 87, 112]. Brain tumors can be distinguished based on behavior, by displaying a "non-malignant" or "malignant" phenotype. Histologically, meningiomas are classified into three subtypes: World Health Organization (WHO) grade I, II, or III. WHO grade I non-malignant (also known as "benign") meningiomas represent the vast majority, encompassing 90 % of cases. WHO grade I meningiomas have a 10-year survival of 70–92 % and a recurrence rate of 7–20 % [23, 51, 65, 96, 112]. WHO grade II (atypical) meningiomas represent 9 % of cases and have a 30–40 % recurrence rate. WHO grade III (anaplastic) meningiomas represent 1 % of cases and have a recurrence rate of 50–80 % [96]. Astrocytomas also display a wide range of histological subtypes, classified as WHO grade I, II, III, or IV tumors. WHO grade I pilocytic astrocytomas occur predominantly in children. WHO grade II diffuse astrocytomas are the most common low-grade intrinsic brain tumor in adults. WHO grade III (anaplastic) and WHO grade IV (glioblastoma) tumors are classified as malignant gliomas. This chapter focuses on adult non-malignant brain tumors with special emphasis on low-grade gliomas (WHO grade II) and benign meningiomas (WHO grade I). Malignant brain tumors are discussed elsewhere in this book.

Low-Grade Gliomas

Low-grade gliomas represent 15 % of all newly diagnosed primary intrinsic brain tumors in adults [26]. Their incidence has increased over the past two decades due to advances in diagnostic imaging and improved diagnostic accuracy [26, 50, 107]. WHO grade II gliomas include diffuse (infiltrative) astrocytoma representing 2.8 % of glioma cases, oligodendrogliomas representing 1.3 % of cases, and mixed oligoastrocytomas representing 1 % of cases [26, 77]. Between 1,500 and

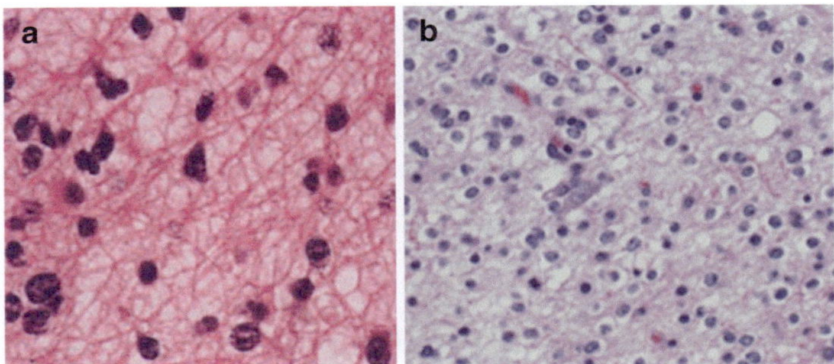

FIGURE 1.1 (**a**) Diffuse astrocytoma demonstrating increased cellularity and disruption of the normal orderly pattern of cells. WHO grade II astrocytomas lack the endothelial proliferation and necrosis seen in malignant gliomas. (**b**) WHO grade II oligodendrogliomas are characterized by uniform circular cells with a halo or "fried egg" appearance

1,800 new low-grade gliomas are diagnosed in the United States each year. Tumor cells infiltrate into brain parenchyma where they can later transform, acquiring more malignant behavior over time. Median time to tumor progression and recurrence is 5.5 years, and median time to malignant transformation is 10.1 years with maximal safe resection. An estimated 50 % of patents with diffuse low-grade gliomas will progress and show recurrence within 5 years of initial diagnosis [32, 79, 85, 105].

The median age at diagnosis for low-grade gliomas is 45 years, with patients ranging from 20 to 70 years of age [26]. Low-grade gliomas are more common among Caucasian men. Histologically, infiltrative astrocytomas display a modest increase in cellularity, disruption of the normal orderly pattern of glial cells, and elongated nuclei (Fig. 1.1). There is no endothelial proliferation or tissue necrosis as is commonly seen in malignant gliomas. Oligodendrogliomas occur predominantly within the gray matter of the cerebral hemispheres, are well-circumscribed, calcified, and have a slight predominance for the frontal lobes. Histologically, oligodendrogliomas are characterized by uniform cell density and round nuclei with perinuclear halos displaying a classic "fried egg" appearance (Fig. 1.1). In 1994, a co-deletion in the long arm of chromosome 1p36 and the short arm of chromosome 19q13 was shown to predict chemosensitivity and better prognosis in patients with low-grade gliomas [57].

Meningiomas

Meningiomas are typically benign, slow-growing extra-axial tumors arising from the arachnoid cap cells of the meninges. They can originate wherever arachnoidal cells are present. They are most commonly located along the falx, cerebral convexity, or sphenoid wing regions. They can also be found at the cerebellopontine angle, choroid plexus, or along the optic nerve [96]. Meningiomas account for 20–37 % of primary brain tumors with an incidence of 7.5 per 100,000 [26, 44, 96]. Meningiomas have one of the largest gender incidence differences, with a female to male ratio of 2:1. Unlike gliomas, African Americans are more commonly affected with meningiomas. Their incidence increases with age, with a median age at diagnosis of 59 years [26].

The vast majority (95–98 %) of meningiomas are WHO grade I or II [26]. Meningiomas are characterized by densely packed sheets of cells, psammoma bodies (whorls of calcium and collagen), intranuclear cytoplasmic pseudo-inclusions, and "Orphan Annie" nuclei (nuclei with central clearing from the peripheral migration of chromatin) (Fig. 1.2).

Risk Factors

The underlying cause of low-grade gliomas in adults is largely unknown and thought to be multifactorial. Though infectious, environmental, immunological, and genetic factors have been implicated, the majority of studies lack large enough study populations to establish causation [86]. The only known modifiable risk factor for the development of low-grade

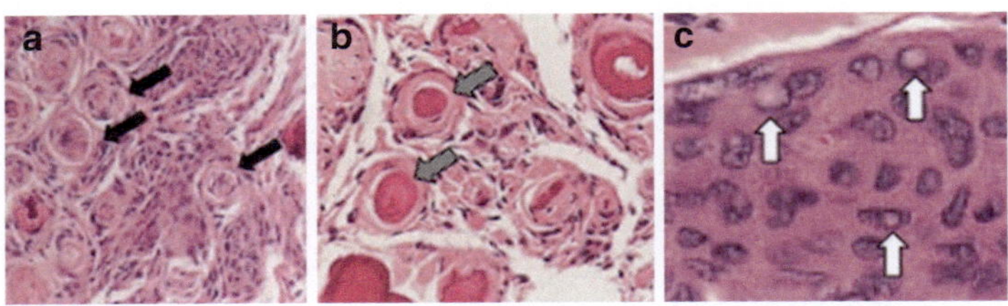

FIGURE 1.2 WHO grade II meningiomas show (**a**) densely packed sheets of cells with whorls (*arrows*), (**b**) calcifications also known as psammoma bodies (*arrows*), and (**c**) cytoplasmic inclusions (*arrows*)

gliomas is prior exposure to ionizing radiation [10]. Though speculative, hereditary factors are not yet known to play a role in low-grade glioma development, although patients with Li-Fraumeni syndrome and neurofibromatosis type 1 have an increased incidence of gliomas and form tumors at a younger age. Genetic studies suggest that point mutations of the tumor suppressor gene *TP53* plays a role in the tumorigenesis of low-grade gliomas. An alteration in tumor metabolism promoting a shift to aerobic glycolysis is a principal step in the development of low-grade gliomas. Isocitrate dehydrogenase (IDH) 1 and 2 catalyze the decarboxylation of isocitrate into alpha ketoglutarate. IDH1 and IDH2 mutations are found in close to 70 % of low-grade gliomas [42, 81, 113]. The impact of these mutations on low-grade diffuse gliomas remains unclear; however, they offer an independent survival benefit in glioma patients regardless of patient age or tumor performance status.

Similar to low-grade gliomas, prior exposure to ionizing radiation is the strongest known risk factor in patients with meningioma [90]. Other modifiable factors that have been studied with inconclusive results include cigarette smoking, exogenous hormone use, personal hair dye use, microwave exposure, prior head trauma, occupational exposures, lead exposure, seasonal allergies, and cell phone use [2, 9, 12, 17, 19, 36, 37, 39, 43, 45, 48, 49, 69, 78, 82, 84, 86, 90, 96, 106]. Neurofibromatosis type 2 (NF2) caused by a mutation on chromosome 22q12 is the most common genetic predisposition associated with meningiomas. Loss of one copy of the NF2 gene occurs in up to 80 % of sporadic meningiomas and all patients with NF2. NF2 patients develop meningiomas at a higher frequency and present earlier in life [96].

Making the Diagnosis

Common Presenting Symptoms

Evaluating patients with non-malignant brain tumors begins with a detailed history. The majority of patients lack symptoms even if there is mass effect. The most common presenting symptoms for patients with low-grade gliomas are seizures (72 %), headaches (30 %), language (7 %), and sensorimotor (32 %) changes [115]. Common presenting symptoms for meningioma patients are seizures (45 %), headaches (34–41 %), dizziness (29.3 %), tinnitus (14.6 %), syncope (9.8 %), memory disturbance (4.9 %), visual disturbance (4.9 %), and trigeminal neuralgia (2.4 %) [51, 68]. Classically, headaches tend to be worse upon waking in the morning and may be severe enough to wake one from sleep. It is not uncommon for tumor-related headaches to initially be misdiagnosed as sinus, tension, or migraine headaches. Headaches related to obstructive hydrocephalus are relatively rare in non-malignant brain tumors; however, this does require urgent neurosurgical evaluation.

Seizures are the most common presenting symptom, occurring in 72–80 % of patients with low-grade gliomas and 45 % of meningioma patients [51, 115]. Seizure control is important for maintaining optimum quality of life. The use of anticonvulsant medications such as levetiracetam, lacosamide, topiramate, or phenytoin in brain tumor patients is somewhat controversial. Patients presenting with seizures should be started on anticonvulsant therapy. However, there is little data to suggest prophylactic use of anticonvulsants to reduce the risk of new-onset seizures in patients with low-grade gliomas or meningiomas [58]. Even so, it is common practice to offer perioperative anticonvulsant medications to patients with large tumors involving highly epileptogenic areas. Gross total resection is the strongest predictor of seizure freedom [30, 88]. Radiotherapy and chemotherapeutic agents such as temozolomide and alkylating agents are also effective in reducing seizure frequency in patients with tumor-associated medication-resistant epilepsy [88].

Physical Findings

The majority of people with non-malignant brain tumors have a normal neurological examination. Physical findings, when evident, are variable depending on tumor location, size, and scope of disease. Papilledema (swelling of the head of the optic nerve associated with engorgement of retinal veins) and oculomotor palsy are due to tumor mass effect and elevated intracranial pressure. Aphasia suggests involvement of cortical or subcortical language centers of the dominant frontal, temporal, or parietal lobes. Focal motor weakness can be caused by tumor invasion of the corticospinal pathway or peritumoral edema, which may be reversible with the administration of corticosteroids. The diagnosis of brain tumor should always be considered in patients who develop a new psychiatric condition.

Symptomatic Versus Asymptomatic Tumors

Non-malignant brain tumors with no clinical symptoms have a different natural history from those that are symptomatic. Incidental low-grade gliomas tend to occur more frequently in females, have smaller tumor volumes, and improved patient outcomes [77, 80]. Incidental low-grade gliomas are more likely to undergo gross total resection; however, if untreated, they demonstrate consistent radiographic growth eventually leading to symptoms over a median of 4 years [76, 77]. Incidental meningiomas fall into one of three growth patterns: no growth, steady linear growth, or exponential growth [68]. For this reason some advocate serial imaging and a brief observation period, reserving surgical intervention for patients with symptomatic lesions, documented tumor growth over time, or imaging suspicious for other pathologic lesions that mimic meningiomas [16].

Imaging

Due to its wide availability, speed, and affordability, non-contrast computed tomography (CT) is commonly the initial imaging modality for symptomatic patients with non-malignant brain tumors. Brain magnetic resonance imaging (MRI) with and without gadolinium contrast is the definitive imaging modality to assess tumor location, size, cellularity, associated cystic components, associated edema or hemorrhage, necrosis, margins and invasion into surrounding structures, vascularity, and enhancement. Radiographically, low-grade gliomas are isodense or hypodense when compared to brain tissue on CT scan and do not enhance with contrast administration. Calcifications are common in oligodendrogliomas. On MRI, low-grade gliomas are isointense to hypointense on T1-weighted imaging, hyperintense on T2-weighted imaging, and are not contrast-enhancing (Fig. 1.3). Meningiomas are hyperintense compared to brain tissue and have a broad dural attachment. On T2-weighted MRI, most meningiomas are hyperintense and are typically contrast-enhancing on both CT and MRI (Fig. 1.4). Radiographic imaging provides information about tumor localization, proximity to functional areas, mass effect, and associated edema [35]. Functional MRI and diffusion tensor imaging (DTI) shows the integrity of white matter tracts and can be used to create an operative corridor or plan for resection that minimizes risk to eloquent surrounding structures (Fig. 1.5). Metabolic MRI or magnetic resonance spectroscopy can be used to supplement information obtained from traditional morphologic MRI, particularly for differentiating radiation necrosis and residual tumor. Cerebral angiography is used preoperatively to illustrate and embolize the vascular supply to meningiomas and hemangiomas (Fig. 1.4c).

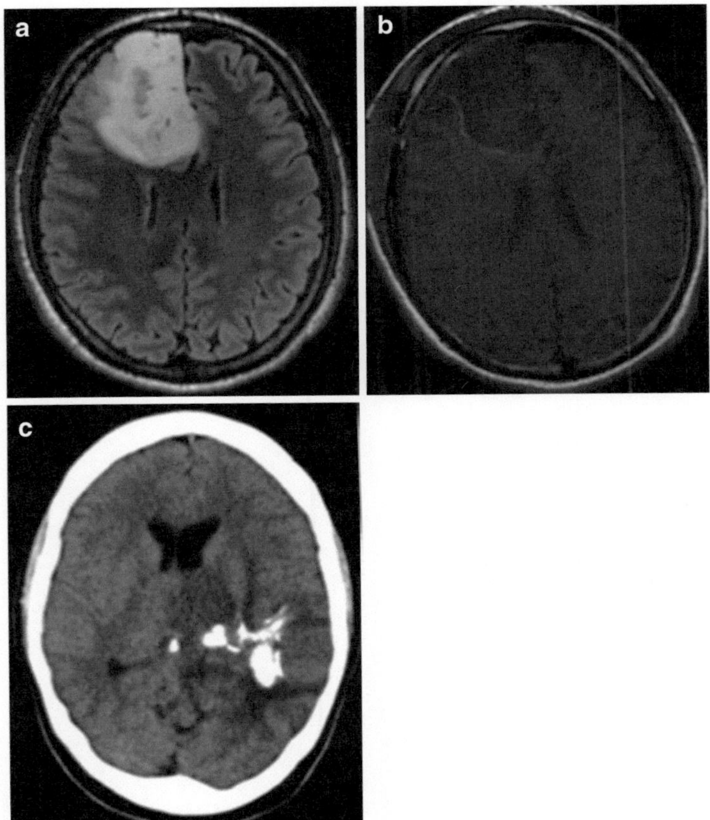

FIGURE 1.3 FLAIR sequence axial MRIs show right frontal diffuse astrocytoma (**a**) before and (**b**) after surgical resection. (**c**) Axial non-contrast head CT shows hyperdensity consistent with calcification typical in oligodendroglioma

Treatment

The decision to offer treatment to patients with non-malignant brain tumors must balance operative risk with the natural history of the tumor and its propensity to transform and grow over time. Mounting evidence places maximal safe surgical resection

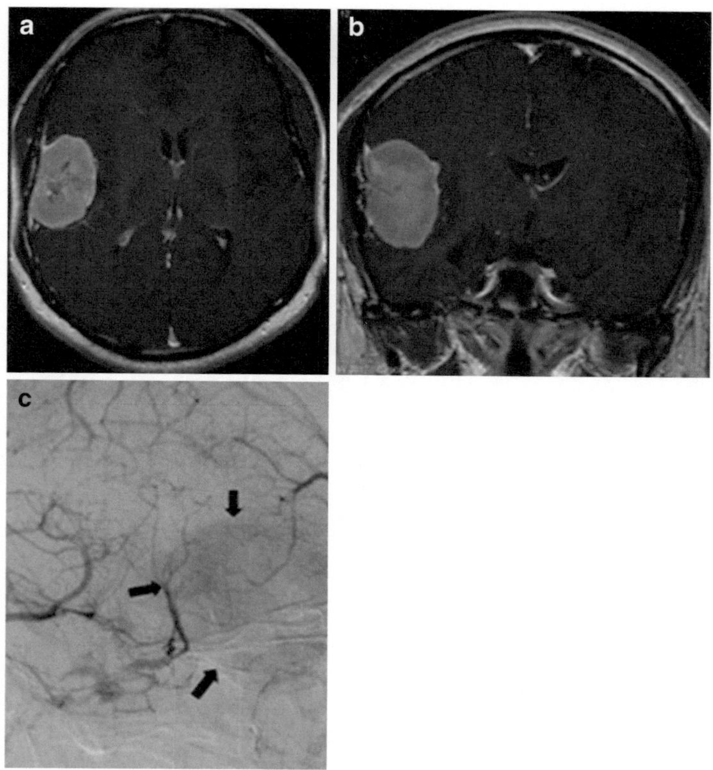

FIGURE 1.4 (**a**) Axial and (**b**) coronal brain MRIs show a broad, contrast-enhancing dural-based lesion consistent with meningioma. (**c**) Cerebral angiography reveals dural feeders to the tumor with a "blush" of vascularity (*arrows*)

alongside patient age, tumor histology, tumor performance status, and molecular markers as predictive of long-term outcome [27, 51, 61, 62, 65, 68, 97, 113]. Corticosteroids such as dexamethasone are commonly used preoperatively to reduce symptoms of mass effect and edema caused by the tumor.

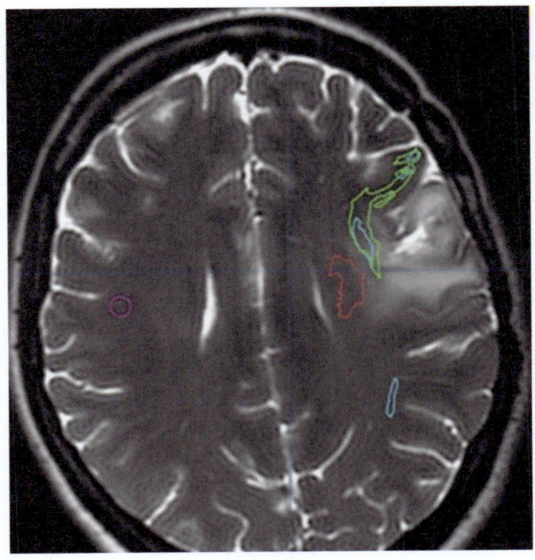

FIGURE 1.5 Axial MRI with DTI shows left frontal tumor. DTI imaging helps identify motor (*red*) and language pathways (*green and blue*) for both preoperative planning and intraoperative navigation

Surgical Considerations and the Value of Extent of Resection

Maximum safe surgical resection is the best option to relieve symptoms, improve functional outcome, and boost long-term survival. Decisions regarding surgical approach require careful consideration of a number of key factors including: tumor size, proximity to presumed functional areas, imaging characteristics, and patient age, health, and functional status. The value of surgical resection for low-grade gliomas has been validated by a number of studies illustrating a survival benefit of 60–90 months with maximal resection [14, 38, 47, 91, 99,

105]. While some advocate initial tumor biopsy followed by watchful waiting for low-grade gliomas, several studies have suggested that this is not the best choice for long-term survival. In a large population-based series of Norwegian patients, early maximal resection was superior to biopsy and watchful waiting with respective 5-year survival rates of 74 and 60 % [47]. Furthermore, maximal resection has also been shown to delay malignant transformation with improved survival and less malignant transformation seen in patients receiving greater than 90 % extent of resection [105]. Tumor-associated epilepsy is also better managed after gross total resection [30, 114]. A small meningioma with no documented growth in an asymptomatic patient can be considered for observation [35]. This however must be balanced with the known fact that younger age at diagnosis and greater extent of resection are strong predictors of improved outcome for meningioma patients [65, 95].

The central goal of brain tumor surgery is maximizing the removal of neoplastic tissue while minimizing collateral damage to functional areas and vascular structures [29]. The timing of surgery is important in preoperative planning. The majority of patients with non-malignant brain tumors can be scheduled for elective surgery. However, patients who present with rapid deterioration due to elevated intracranial pressure or obstructive hydrocephalus require prompt intervention. For low-grade gliomas, the goal is to safely remove as much tumor as possible, as visualized by T2/FLAIR signal. The goal for meningioma resection is to remove both the tumor and its dural origin. A variety of technologies have been developed to improve surgical outcomes. Stereotactic navigation (also known as neuronavigation) is utilized to precisely localize tumor location and tailor focused craniotomies, but there is little evidence that it can improve extent of resection. Intraoperative MRI, an approach in which brain tumor resection is performed in a highly specialized surgical suite containing MRI, is another technique used to improve identification of residual tumor [59, 63, 71, 98]. The use of direct stimulation mapping to identify functional

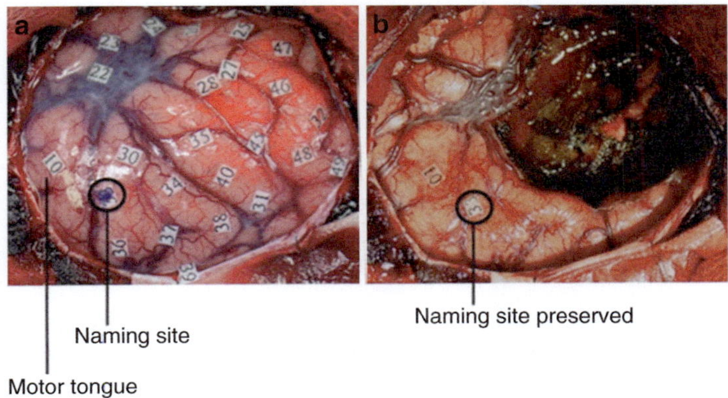

FIGURE 1.6 (**a**) Intraoperative stimulation testing allows for the identification of language, sensory, and motor sites. Numbered markers are placed 1 cm apart for testing of speech arrest, naming, and reading. (**b**) After tumor removal, functional sites remain intact

pathways is the gold standard for preserving language and sensorimotor function. Individual patient variability and pathway distortion by mass lesions makes localization of functional sites difficult by any other means [5, 18, 28, 40, 54, 72–74, 92, 102] (Fig. 1.6). Numerous studies have failed to predict the specific location of language sites using anatomical locations and functional neuroimaging (DTI and functional MRI) [1, 21, 31, 41, 60, 67, 83, 101, 110]. Using specialized neuroanesthesia, awake brain tumor surgery has proven both safe and effective, with an acceptable morbidity and mortality compared with asleep procedures [6, 22, 34, 55, 56, 89, 92, 94, 109].

Following brain tumor surgery, patients are commonly observed closely in an intensive care setting with hemodynamic and neurological monitoring. Corticosteroid medications are tapered and anticonvulsants continued in patients who have a seizure history. Given the prognostic significance of extent of resection, it is standard practice for many surgeons to obtain an early postoperative MRI to evaluate for residual tumor.

Adjuvant Therapies

Although surgical resection is the foundation of brain tumor therapy, it is incapable of eliminating every tumor cell. Adjuvant radiation and chemotherapeutic regimens have been developed to treat remaining tumor cells.

Radiation

Radiation therapy can be used for select patients with recurrent low-grade gliomas to improve progression-free survival [111]. Radiation causes damage to cellular structures, inducing lethal mutations in cellular DNA and activating pathways for programmed cell death. External beam radiation can be delivered to a small precise location in a single treatment (stereotactic radiosurgery [SRS]), or in an interrupted manner (fractionated radiotherapy) that allows for repair of normal tissue between treatments. Factors that influence the use of radiation therapy include patient age (often avoided in younger patients given neurocognitive risks), speed of recurrence, volume of residual tumor after surgery, and a tumor's molecular markers such as chromosomal translations at 1p and 19q (used to identify oligodendrogliomas, which are more sensitive to chemotherapy and radiation) [20, 46]. There is little benefit to higher doses of fractionated radiotherapy for low-grade gliomas (>45 Gy) [53]. One must balance the benefits of radiation therapy with potential late neurocognitive toxicities [4].

For convexity meningiomas, complete surgical resection of the tumor and dural attachment is often feasible. In contrast however, complete resection is often not possible for large skull-base meningiomas involving areas with high morbidity (cavernous sinus, petroclival region, optic nerve sheath, etc.). External beam radiotherapy should be considered as a safe adjuvant to surgery [93]. Long-term studies comparing adjuvant radiation with observation in patients with large skull-base meningiomas have demonstrated better tumor control after radiation therapy with 5-, 10-, and 15-year survival rates of 79–98 %, 68–93 %, and 92 %, respectively, and low morbidity (3.6 %) [24, 33, 64]. Intensity modulated radiation therapy and SRS therapy are additional options to external beam radiation for recurrent or partially resected meningiomas in patients for whom surgery is not an option.

Chemotherapy

The role of chemotherapy for non-malignant brain tumors remains unclear. Several studies exploring the use of temozolomide or procarbizine, carmustine, and vincristine (PCV) immediately after surgical resection showed little clinical efficacy [11, 13]. However, in select patients with 1p19q deletions and oligodendroglial lineage, the evidence suggests better seizure control, a progression-free survival benefit, and improved quality of life with sensitivity to PCV and temozolomide [11, 75, 77]. There is preliminary data proposing the utility of neoadjuvant temozolomide to reduce tumor volume before surgery, thereby allowing for maximal safe surgical resection [7, 8]. Chemotherapeutic agents have thus far failed to show clinical efficacy in recurrent meningioma [103]. Possible exceptions to this are currently under investigation including hydroxyurea (71 % of patients with stable disease after 2 years) and a multidrug regimen of cyclophosphamide, doxorubicin, and vincristine [15, 70, 100]. Numerous clinical trials are currently underway testing the efficacy of targeting therapies against molecular signaling pathways known to be up-regulated in non-malignant brain tumors. One promising example of this involves the use of everolimus against the AKT-mTOR pathway for patients with low-grade gliomas.

Prognosis and Long-Term Outcome

Several factors are known to be predictive of outcome for patients with non-malignant brain tumors. Negative prognostic factors for patients with low-grade gliomas include age greater than 40 years, tumor diameter greater than 4 cm,

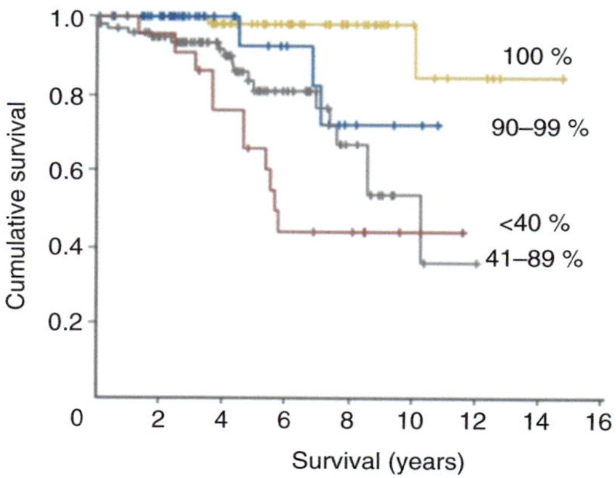

FIGURE 1.7 Survival curves for total, subtotal, and partial resections for low-grade gliomas (Adapted with permission [105])

astrocytoma or oligoastrocytoma histology, tumors crossing the midline, and patients with greater than 1 cm^3 of residual tumor after surgery [52, 53, 91]. These patients have a higher incidence of tumor recurrence. Patients with low-grade gliomas have a median survival ranging between 4.6 and 9.8 years and median time to malignant progression of 8.8–11.4 years when extent of resection is greater than 90 % [3, 14, 105]. Furthermore, patients with at least 90 % extent of resection have 5- and 8-year survival rates of 76 and 60 %, respectively [105] (Fig. 1.7).

The prognosis for meningioma patients is determined by the extent of surgical resection, patient age at diagnosis, and tumor grade (WHO grade I). The Simpson grading system was developed as a predictive model of 10-year recurrence based on extent of resection. Macroscopic gross total resection with excision of affected dura and bone (grade 1) offers a 9 % 10-year recurrence rate. Macroscopic gross total resection with coagulation of attached dura (grade 2) offers a 10-year recurrence rate of 19 %. Macroscopic resection without resection or coagulation of affected dura (grade 3) offers a 10-year recurrence rate of 29 %. Subtotal resection and biopsies (grades 4 and 5) offer 10-year recurrences of greater than 40 % [96, 104]. Five-year survival rates of 70–92 % and 10-year survival rates of 80–86 % have been demonstrated in patients with WHO grade I meningiomas [66, 95, 108]. Recurrence has been estimated to occur in approximately 20 % of patients with benign meningiomas but is much more common in WHO grade II and III tumors.

Conclusions

Non-malignant brain tumors are a fairly common diagnosis, and patients can live for decades after treatment. Low-grade gliomas are slow-growing tumors originating from supporting glial cells, while meningiomas grow attached to dural surfaces outside of the brain. Prior radiation exposure is the only known risk factor. Surgical resection plays a critical role. Maximal safe resection using techniques such as neuronavigation, functional MRI, DTI, and stimulation mapping allow for preservation of neurological function while reducing tumor burden. Subsequent radiotherapy can improve progression-free survival for recurrent tumors and residual disease. Targeted chemotherapeutic agents against specific pathways necessary for tumor growth are currently being investigated.

References

1. Alexander AL, Lee JE, Lazar M, Field AS. Diffusion tensor imaging of the brain. Neurotherapeutics. 2007;4(3):316–29.
2. Barnholtz-Sloan JS, Kruchko C. Meningiomas: causes and risk factors. Neurosurg Focus. 2007;23(4):E2.
3. Bauman G, Fisher B, Watling C, Cairncross JG, Macdonald D. Adult supratentorial low-grade glioma: long-term experience at a single institution. Int J Radiat Oncol Biol Phys. 2009;75(5):1401–7.
4. Baumert BG, Stupp R. Low-grade glioma: a challenge in therapeutic options: the role of radiotherapy. Ann Oncol. 2008;19(7):vii217–22.

5. Berger MS. Lesions in functional ("eloquent") cortex and subcortical white matter. Clin Neurosurg. 1994;41:444–63.
6. Blanshard HJ, Chung F, Manninen PH, Taylor MD, Bernstein M. Awake craniotomy for removal of intracranial tumor: considerations for early discharge. Anesth Analg. 2001;92(1):89–94.
7. Blonski M, Pallud J, Goze C, Mandonnet E, Rigau V, Bauchet L, et al. Neoadjuvant chemotherapy may optimize the extent of resection of World Health Organization grade II gliomas: a case series of 17 patients. J Neurooncol. 2013;113(2):267–75.
8. Blonski M, Taillandier L, Herbet G, Maldonado IL, Beauchesne P, Fabbro M, et al. Combination of neoadjuvant chemotherapy followed by surgical resection as a new strategy for WHO grade II gliomas: a study of cognitive status and quality of life. J Neurooncol. 2012;106(2):353–66.
9. Bluhm EC, Zahm SH, Fine HA, Black PM, Loeffler JS, Shapiro WR, et al. Personal hair dye use and risks of glioma, meningioma, and acoustic neuroma among adults. Am J Epidemiol. 2007;165(1):63–71.
10. Bondy ML, Scheurer ME, Malmer B, Barnholtz-Sloan JS, Davis FG, Il'yasova D, et al. Brain tumor epidemiology: consensus from the Brain Tumor Epidemiology Consortium. Cancer. 2008;113(7 Suppl):1953–68.
11. Brada M, Viviers L, Abson C, Hines F, Britton J, Ashley S, et al. Phase II study of primary temozolomide chemotherapy in patients with WHO grade II gliomas. Ann Oncol. 2003;14(12): 1715–21.
12. Brenner AV, Linet MS, Fine HA, Shapiro WR, Selker RG, Black PM, et al. History of allergies and autoimmune diseases and risk of brain tumors in adults. Int J Cancer. 2002;99(2):252–9.
13. Buckner JC, Gesme Jr D, O'Fallon JR, Hammack JE, Stafford S, Brown PD, et al. Phase II trial of procarbazine, lomustine, and vincristine as initial therapy for patients with low-grade oligodendroglioma or oligoastrocytoma: efficacy and associations with chromosomal abnormalities. J Clin Oncol. 2003;21(2):251–5.
14. Capelle L, Fontaine D, Mandonnet E, Taillandier L, Golmard JL, Bauchet L, et al. Spontaneous and therapeutic prognostic factors in adult hemispheric World Health Organization Grade II gliomas: a series of 1097 cases: clinical article. J Neurosurg. 2013;118(6):1157–68.
15. Chamberlain MC. Adjuvant combined modality therapy for malignant meningiomas. J Neurosurg. 1996;84(5):733–6.
16. Chamoun R, Krisht KM, Couldwell WT. Incidental meningiomas. Neurosurg Focus. 2011;31(6):E19.

17. Claus EB, Black PM, Bondy ML, Calvocoressi L, Schildkraut JM, Wiemels JL, et al. Exogenous hormone use and meningioma risk: what do we tell our patients? Cancer. 2007;110(3):471–6.
18. Coello AF, Moritz-Gasser S, Martino J, Martinoni M, Matsuda R, Duffau H. Selection of intraoperative tasks for awake mapping based on relationships between tumor location and functional networks. J Neurosurg. 2013;119(6):1380–94.
19. Custer B, Longstreth Jr WT, Phillips LE, Koepsell TD, Van Belle G. Hormonal exposures and the risk of intracranial meningioma in women: a population-based case-control study. BMC Cancer. 2006;6:152.
20. Daniels TB, Brown PD, Felten SJ, Wu W, Buckner JC, Arusell RM, et al. Validation of EORTC prognostic factors for adults with low-grade glioma: a report using intergroup 86-72-51. Int J Radiat Oncol Biol Phys. 2011;81(1):218–24.
21. Davies KG, Maxwell RE, Jennum P, Dhuna A, Beniak TE, Destafney E, et al. Language function following subdural grid-directed temporal lobectomy. Acta Neurol Scand. 1994;90(3):201–6.
22. De Benedictis A, Moritz-Gasser S, Duffau H. Awake mapping optimizes the extent of resection for low-grade gliomas in eloquent areas. Neurosurgery. 2010;66(6):1074–84.
23. DeAngelis LM. Brain tumors. N Engl J Med. 2001;344(2): 114–23.
24. Debus J, Wuendrich M, Pirzkal A, Hoess A, Schlegel W, Zuna I, et al. High efficacy of fractionated stereotactic radiotherapy of large base-of-skull meningiomas: long-term results. J Clin Oncol. 2001;19(15):3547–53.
25. Deorah S, Lynch CF, Sibenaller ZA, Ryken TC. Trends in brain cancer incidence and survival in the United States: Surveillance, Epidemiology, and End Results Program, 1973 to 2001. Neurosurg Focus. 2006;20(4):E1.
26. Dolecek TA, Propp JM, Stroup NE, Kruchko C. CBTRUS statistical report: primary brain and central nervous system tumors diagnosed in the United States in 2005-2009. Neuro Oncol. 2012;14 Suppl 5:v1–49.
27. Duffau H. Surgery of low-grade gliomas: towards a 'functional neurooncology'. Curr Opin Oncol. 2009;21(6):543–9.
28. Duffau H. The huge plastic potential of adult brain and the role of connectomics: new insights provided by serial mappings in glioma surgery. Cortex. 2013;19(13):00207–4.
29. Duffau H, Mandonnet E. The "onco-functional balance" in surgery for diffuse low-grade glioma: integrating the extent of

resection with quality of life. Acta Neurochir. 2013;155(6):951–7.

30. Englot DJ, Han SJ, Berger MS, Barbaro NM, Chang EF. Extent of surgical resection predicts seizure freedom in low-grade temporal lobe brain tumors. Neurosurgery. 2012;70(4):921–8.

31. FitzGerald DB, Cosgrove GR, Ronner S, Jiang H, Buchbinder BR, Belliveau JW, et al. Location of language in the cortex: a comparison between functional MR imaging and electrocortical stimulation. AJNR Am J Neuroradiol. 1997;18(8):1529–39.

32. Frazier JL, Johnson MW, Burger PC, Weingart JD, Quinones-Hinojosa A. Rapid malignant transformation of low-grade astrocytomas: report of 2 cases and review of the literature. World Neurosurg. 2010;73(1):53–62.

33. Goldsmith BJ, Wara WM, Wilson CB, Larson DA. Postoperative irradiation for subtotally resected meningiomas. A retrospective analysis of 140 patients treated from 1967 to 1990. J Neurosurg. 1994;80(2):195–201.

34. Grossman R, Nossek E, Sitt R, Hayat D, Shahar T, Barzilai O, et al. Outcome of elderly patients undergoing awake-craniotomy for tumor resection. Ann Surg Oncol. 2013;20(5):1722–8.

35. Hallinan JT, Hegde AN, Lim WE. Dilemmas and diagnostic difficulties in meningioma. Clin Radiol. 2013;68(8):837–44.

36. Hardell L, Carlberg M, Hansson MK. Pooled analysis of two case-control studies on use of cellular and cordless telephones and the risk for malignant brain tumours diagnosed in 1997-2003. Int Arch Occup Environ Health. 2006;79(8):630–9.

37. Hardell L, Hallquist A, Mild KH, Carlberg M, Pahlson A, Lilja A. Cellular and cordless telephones and the risk for brain tumours. Eur J Cancer Prev. 2002;11(4):377–86.

38. Hardesty DA, Sanai N. The value of glioma extent of resection in the modern neurosurgical era. Front Neurol. 2012;3:140.

39. Hatch EE, Linet MS, Zhang J, Fine HA, Shapiro WR, Selker RG, et al. Reproductive and hormonal factors and risk of brain tumors in adult females. Int J Cancer. 2005;114(5):797–805.

40. Herholz K, Thiel A, Wienhard K, Pietrzyk U, von Stockhausen HM, Karbe H, et al. Individual functional anatomy of verb generation. Neuroimage. 1996;3(3 Pt 1):185–94.

41. Hirsch J, Ruge MI, Kim KH, Correa DD, Victor JD, Relkin NR, et al. An integrated functional magnetic resonance imaging procedure for preoperative mapping of cortical areas associated with tactile, motor, language, and visual functions. Neurosurgery. 2000;47(3):711–21.

42. Houillier C, Wang X, Kaloshi G, Mokhtari K, Guillevin R, Laffaire J, et al. IDH1 or IDH2 mutations predict longer survival and response to temozolomide in low-grade gliomas. Neurology. 2010;75(17):1560–6.

43. Hu J, Little J, Xu T, Zhao X, Guo L, Jia X, et al. Risk factors for meningioma in adults: a case-control study in northeast China. Int J Cancer. 1999;83(3):299–304.

44. Ibebuike K, Ouma J, Gopal R. Meningiomas among intracranial neoplasms in Johannesburg, South Africa: prevalence, clinical observations and review of the literature. Afr Health Sci. 2013;13(1):118–21.

45. Inskip PD, Tarone RE, Hatch EE, Wilcosky TC, Shapiro WR, Selker RG, et al. Cellular-telephone use and brain tumors. N Engl J Med. 2001;344(2):79–86.

46. Iwadate Y, Matsutani T, Hasegawa Y, Shinozaki N, Higuchi Y, Saeki N. Favorable long-term outcome of low-grade oligodendrogliomas irrespective of 1p/19q status when treated without radiotherapy. J Neurooncol. 2011;102(3):443–9.

47. Jakola AS, Myrmel KS, Kloster R, Torp SH, Lindal S, Unsgard G, et al. Comparison of a strategy favoring early surgical resection vs a strategy favoring watchful waiting in low-grade gliomas. JAMA. 2012;308(18):1881–8.

48. Jhawar BS, Fuchs CS, Colditz GA, Stampfer MJ. Sex steroid hormone exposures and risk for meningioma. J Neurosurg. 2003;99(5):848–53.

49. Johansen C, Boice Jr J, McLaughlin J, Olsen J. Cellular telephones and cancer–a nationwide cohort study in Denmark. J Natl Cancer Inst. 2001;93(3):203–7.

50. Jukich PJ, McCarthy BJ, Surawicz TS, Freels S, Davis FG. Trends in incidence of primary brain tumors in the United States, 1985-1994. Neuro Oncol. 2001;3(3):141–51.

51. Kallio M, Sankila R, Hakulinen T, Jaaskelainen J. Factors affecting operative and excess long-term mortality in 935 patients with intracranial meningioma. Neurosurgery. 1992;31(1):2–12.

52. Karim AB, Afra D, Cornu P, Bleehan N, Schraub S, De Witte O, et al. Randomized trial on the efficacy of radiotherapy for cerebral low-grade glioma in the adult: European Organization for Research and Treatment of Cancer Study 22845 with the Medical Research Council study BRO4: an interim analysis. Int J Radiat Oncol Biol Phys. 2002;52(2):316–24.

53. Karim AB, Maat B, Hatlevoll R, Menten J, Rutten EH, Thomas DG, et al. A randomized trial on dose-response in radiation

therapy of low-grade cerebral glioma: European Organization for Research and Treatment of Cancer (EORTC) Study 22844. Int J Radiat Oncol Biol Phys. 1996;36(3):549–56.

54. Keles GE, Lundin DA, Lamborn KR, Chang EF, Ojemann G, Berger MS. Intraoperative subcortical stimulation mapping for hemispherical perirolandic gliomas located within or adjacent to the descending motor pathways: evaluation of morbidity and assessment of functional outcome in 294 patients. J Neurosurg. 2004;100(3):369–75.

55. Khu KJ, Doglietto F, Radovanovic I, Taleb F, Mendelsohn D, Zadeh G, et al. Patients' perceptions of awake and outpatient craniotomy for brain tumor: a qualitative study. J Neurosurg. 2010;112(5):1056–60.

56. Kim SS, McCutcheon IE, Suki D, Weinberg JS, Sawaya R, Lang FF, et al. Awake craniotomy for brain tumors near eloquent cortex: correlation of intraoperative cortical mapping with neurological outcomes in 309 consecutive patients. Neurosurgery. 2009;64(5):836–45.

57. Kleihues P, Soylemezoglu F, Schauble B, Scheithauer BW, Burger PC. Histopathology, classification, and grading of gliomas. Glia. 1995;15(3):211–21.

58. Komotar RJ, Raper DM, Starke RM, Iorgulescu JB, Gutin PH. Prophylactic antiepileptic drug therapy in patients undergoing supratentorial meningioma resection: a systematic analysis of efficacy. J Neurosurg. 2011;115(3):483–90.

59. Kowalik K, Truwit C, Hall W, Kucharczyk J. Initial assessment of costs and benefits of MRI-guided brain tumor resection. Eur Radiol. 2000;10(3):S366–7.

60. Krieg SM, Buchmann NH, Gempt J, Shiban E, Meyer B, Ringel F. Diffusion tensor imaging fiber tracking using navigated brain stimulation–a feasibility study. Acta Neurochir. 2012;154(3):555–63.

61. Lacroix M, Abi-Said D, Fourney DR, Gokaslan ZL, Shi W, DeMonte F, et al. A multivariate analysis of 416 patients with glioblastoma multiforme: prognosis, extent of resection, and survival. J Neurosurg. 2001;95(2):190–8.

62. Lote K, Egeland T, Hager B, Stenwig B, Skullerud K, Berg-Johnsen J, et al. Survival, prognostic factors, and therapeutic efficacy in low-grade glioma: a retrospective study in 379 patients. J Clin Oncol. 1997;15(9):3129–40.

63. Lu J, Wu J, Yao C, Zhuang D, Qiu T, Hu X, et al. Awake language mapping and 3-Tesla intraoperative MRI-guided volumetric

resection for gliomas in language areas. J Clin Neurosci. 2013;20(9):1280–7.

64. Marta GN, Correa SF, Teixeira MJ. Meningioma: review of the literature with emphasis on the approach to radiotherapy. Expert Rev Anticancer Ther. 2011;11(11):1749–58.

65. McCarthy BJ, Davis FG, Freels S, Surawicz TS, Damek DM, Grutsch J, et al. Factors associated with survival in patients with meningioma. J Neurosurg. 1998;88(5):831–9.

66. Mirimanoff RO, Dosoretz DE, Linggood RM, Ojemann RG, Martuza RL. Meningioma: analysis of recurrence and progression following neurosurgical resection. J Neurosurg. 1985;62(1):18–24.

67. Mueller WM, Yetkin FZ, Hammeke TA, Morris 3rd GL, Swanson SJ, Reichert K, et al. Functional magnetic resonance imaging mapping of the motor cortex in patients with cerebral tumors. Neurosurgery. 1996;39(3):515–20.

68. Nakamura M, Roser F, Michel J. Jacobs C, Samii M. The natural history of incidental meningiomas. Neurosurgery. 2003;53(1):62–70.

69. Navas-Acien A, Pollan M, Gustavsson P, Plato N. Occupation, exposure to chemicals and risk of gliomas and meningiomas in Sweden. Am J Ind Med. 2002;42(3):214–27.

70. Newton HB, Slivka MA, Stevens C. Hydroxyurea chemotherapy for unresectable or residual meningioma. J Neurooncol. 2000;49(2):165–70.

71. Nimsky C, Ganslandt O, Tomandl B, Buchfelder M, Fahlbusch R. Low-field magnetic resonance imaging for intraoperative use in neurosurgery: a 5-year experience. Eur Radiol. 2002;12(11):2690–703.

72. Ojemann G, Ojemann J, Lettich E, Berger M. Cortical language localization in left, dominant hemisphere. An electrical stimulation mapping investigation in 117 patients. J Neurosurg. 1989;71(3):316–26.

73. Ojemann GA. Cortical organization of language. J Neurosci. 1991;11(8):2281–7.

74. Ojemann GA, Whitaker HA. Language localization and variability. Brain Lang. 1978;6(2):239–60.

75. Pace A, Vidiri A, Galie E, Carosi M, Telera S, Cianciulli AM, et al. Temozolomide chemotherapy for progressive low-grade glioma: clinical benefits and radiological response. Ann Oncol. 2003;14(12):1722–6.

76. Pallud J, Blonski M, Mandonnet E, Audureau E, Fontaine D, Sanai N, et al. Velocity of tumor spontaneous expansion predicts

24   S.L. Hervey-Jumper and M.S. Berger

long-term outcomes for diffuse low-grade gliomas. Neuro Oncol. 2013;15(5):595–606.

77. Pallud J, Fontaine D, Duffau H, Mandonnet E, Sanai N, Taillandier L, et al. Natural history of incidental World Health Organization grade II gliomas. Ann Neurol. 2010;68(5):727–33.

78. Phillips LE, Longstreth Jr WT, Koepsell T, Custer BS, Kukull WA, van Belle G. Active and passive cigarette smoking and risk of intracranial meningioma. Neuroepidemiology. 2005;24(3):117–22.

79. Piepmeier J, Christopher S, Spencer D, Byrne T, Kim J, Knisel JP, et al. Variations in the natural history and survival of patients with supratentorial low-grade astrocytomas. Neurosurgery. 1996;38(5):872–8.

80. Potts MB, Smith JS, Molinaro AM, Berger MS. Natural history and surgical management of incidentally discovered low-grade gliomas. J Neurosurg. 2012;116(2):365–72.

81. Prensner JR, Chinnaiyan AM. Metabolism unhinged: IDH mutations in cancer. Nat Med. 2011;17(3):291–3.

82. Preston-Martin S, Mack W, Henderson BE. Risk factors for gliomas and meningiomas in males in Los Angeles County. Cancer Res. 1989;49(21):6137–43.

83. Quinones-Hinojosa A, Ojemann SG, Sanai N, Dillon WP, Berger MS. Preoperative correlation of intraoperative cortical mapping with magnetic resonance imaging landmarks to predict localization of the Broca area. J Neurosurg. 2003;99(2):311–8.

84. Rajaraman P, Stewart PA, Samet JM, Schwartz BS, Linet MS, Zahm SH, et al. Lead, genetic susceptibility, and risk of adult brain tumors. Cancer Epidemiol Biomarkers Prev. 2006;15(12):2514–20.

85. Recht LD, Lew R, Smith TW. Suspected low-grade glioma: is deferring treatment safe? Ann Neurol. 1992;31(4):431–6.

86. Repacholi MH, Lerchl A, Roosli M, Sienkiewicz Z, Auvinen A, Breckenkamp J, et al. Systematic review of wireless phone use and brain cancer and other head tumors. Bioelectromagnetics. 2012;33(3):187–206.

87. Rigau V, Zouaoui S, Mathieu-Daude H, Darlix A, Maran A, Tretarre B, et al. French brain tumor database: 5-year histological results on 25 756 cases. Brain Pathol. 2011;21(6):633–44.

88. Ruda R, Bello L, Duffau H, Soffietti R. Seizures in low-grade gliomas: natural history, pathogenesis, and outcome after treatments. Neuro Oncol. 2012;14 Suppl 4:iv55–64.

89. Sacko O, Lauwers-Cances V, Brauge D, Sesay M, Brenner A, Roux FE. Awake craniotomy vs surgery under general anesthesia for resection of supratentorial lesions. Neurosurgery. 2011; 68(5):1192–8.

90. Sadetzki S, Flint-Richter P, Ben-Tal T, Nass D. Radiation-induced meningioma: a descriptive study of 253 cases. J Neurosurg. 2002;97(5):1078–82.

91. Sanai N, Berger MS. Glioma extent of resection and its impact on patient outcome. Neurosurgery. 2008;62(4):753–64.

92. Sanai N, Berger MS. Operative techniques for gliomas and the value of extent of resection. Neurotherapeutics. 2009;6(3):478–86.

93. Sanai N, Chang S, Berger MS. Low-grade gliomas in adults. J Neurosurg. 2011;115(5):948–65.

94. Sanai N, Mirzadeh Z, Berger MS. Functional outcome after language mapping for glioma resection. N Engl J Med. 2008;358(1):18–27.

95. Sankila R, Kallio M, Jaaskelainen J, Hakulinen T. Long-term survival of 1986 patients with intracranial meningioma diagnosed from 1953 to 1984 in Finland. Comparison of the observed and expected survival rates in a population-based series. Cancer. 1992;70(6):1568–76.

96. Saraf S, McCarthy BJ, Villano JL. Update on meningiomas. Oncologist. 2011;16(11):1604–13.

97. Scerrati M, Roselli R, Iacoangeli M, Pompucci A, Rossi GF. Prognostic factors in low grade (WHO grade II) gliomas of the cerebral hemispheres: the role of surgery. J Neurol Neurosurg Psychiatry. 1996;61(3):291–6.

98. Schneider JP, Schulz T, Schmidt F, Dietrich J, Lieberenz S, Trantakis C, et al. Gross-total surgery of supratentorial low-grade gliomas under intraoperative MR guidance. AJNR Am J Neuroradiol. 2001;22(1):89–98.

99. Schomas DA, Laack NN, Rao RD, Meyer FB, Shaw EG, O'Neill BP, et al. Intracranial low-grade gliomas in adults: 30-year experience with long-term follow-up at Mayo Clinic. Neuro Oncol. 2009;11(4):437–45.

100. Schrell UM, Rittig MG, Anders M, Koch UH, Marschalek R, Kiesewetter F, et al. Hydroxyurea for treatment of unresectable and recurrent meningiomas. II. Decrease in the size of meningiomas in patients treated with hydroxyurea. J Neurosurg. 1997;86(5):840–4.

101. Seghier ML, Lazeyras F, Pegna AJ, Annoni JM, Zimine I, Mayer E, et al. Variability of fMRI activation during a phonological and semantic language task in healthy subjects. Hum Brain Mapp. 2004;23(3):140–55.

102. Seitz RJ, Huang Y, Knorr U, Tellmann L, Herzog H, Freund HJ. Large-scale plasticity of the human motor cortex. Neuroreport. 1995;6(5):742–4.

103. Sherman WJ, Raizer JJ. Chemotherapy: what is its role in meningioma? Expert Rev Neurother. 2012;12(10):1189–95.
104. Simpson D. The recurrence of intracranial meningiomas after surgical treatment. J Neurol Neurosurg Psychiatry. 1957;20(1):22–39.
105. Smith JS, Chang EF, Lamborn KR, Chang SM, Prados MD, Cha S, et al. Role of extent of resection in the long-term outcome of low-grade hemispheric gliomas. J Clin Oncol. 2008;26(8):1338–45.
106. Steenland K, Boffetta P. Lead and cancer in humans: where are we now? Am J Ind Med. 2000;38(3):295–9.
107. Stieber VW. Low-grade gliomas. Curr Treat Options Oncol. 2001;2(6):495–506.
108. Talback M, Stenbeck M, Rosen M. Up-to-date long-term survival of cancer patients: an evaluation of period analysis on Swedish Cancer Registry data. Eur J Cancer. 2004;40(9):1361–72.
109. Taylor MD, Bernstein M. Awake craniotomy with brain mapping as the routine surgical approach to treating patients with supratentorial intraaxial tumors: a prospective trial of 200 cases. J Neurosurg. 1999;90(1):35–41.
110. Tzourio-Mazoyer N, Josse G, Crivello F, Mazoyer B. Interindividual variability in the hemispheric organization for speech. Neuroimage. 2004;21(1):422–35.
111. van den Bent MJ, Afra D, de Witte O, Ben Hassel M, Schraub S, Hoang-Xuan K, et al. Long-term efficacy of early versus delayed radiotherapy for low-grade astrocytoma and oligodendroglioma in adults: the EORTC 22845 randomised trial. Lancet. 2005;366(9490):985–90.
112. Vranic A, Peyre M, Kalamarides M. New insights into meningioma: from genetics to trials. Curr Opin Oncol. 2012;24(6):660–5.
113. Yan H, Parsons DW, Jin G, McLendon R, Rasheed BA, Yuan W, et al. IDH1 and IDH2 mutations in gliomas. N Engl J Med. 2009;360(8):765–73.
114. You G, Sha ZY, Yan W, Zhang W, Wang YZ, Li SW, et al. Seizure characteristics and outcomes in 508 Chinese adult patients undergoing primary resection of low-grade gliomas: a clinicopathological study. Neuro Oncol. 2012;14(2):230–41.
115. Youland RS, Schomas DA, Brown PD, Nwachukwu C, Buckner JC, Giannini C, et al. Changes in presentation, treatment, and outcomes of adult low-grade gliomas over the past fifty years. Neuro Oncol. 2013;15(8):1102–10.

Chapter 2
Malignant Brain Tumors

Leonardo Rangel-Castilla and Robert F. Spetzler

Primary malignant tumors of the central nervous system (CNS) are infrequent, occurring at a rate of about 4 per 100,000 persons. The cause of primary malignant brain tumors is not yet well understood. They result from a combination of genetic predisposition and environmental factors such as therapeutic brain radiation. However, secondary malignant tumors—metastatic tumors—are by far the most common type of malignant lesions in the CNS. The lung, breast, colon, and skin are the most common sites of primary origin, but metastatic tumors can develop from almost anywhere in the body [5].

In 2007, the World Health Organization (WHO) classified all benign and malignant brain tumors into nine groups. Tumors of the neuroepithelial tissue, which are called gliomas, represent the largest group (50–60 %) [3]. They can be divided into the subgroups astrocytic, oligodendroglial, mixed, ependymal, choroid plexus, neuronal, mixed neuronal-glial, neuroblastic, pineal, and embryonal tumors. The largest of these subgroups is the astrocytic tumors, also called astrocytomas. In general, they are poorly demarcated and infiltrate

L. Rangel-Castilla, MD • R.F. Spetzler, MD (✉)
Division of Neurological Surgery, c/o Neuroscience Publications,
Barrow Neurological Institute, St. Joseph's Hospital and Medical
Center, 350 W. Thomas Road, Phoenix, AZ 85013, USA
e-mail: neuropub@dignityhealth.org; robert.spetzler@bnaneuro.net

A. Agrawal, G. Britz (eds.), *Emergency Approaches to Neurosurgical Conditions*, DOI 10.1007/978-3-319-10693-9_2,
© Springer International Publishing Switzerland 2015

the adjacent brain tissue diffusely. Pilocytic astrocytomas (WHO grade I) are seen mainly in children and have a relatively good prognosis. Low-grade diffuse astrocytomas (WHO grade II) are usually slow-growing tumors. Anaplastic astrocytomas (WHO grade III) are also relatively slow-growing tumors with greater cellularity. Glioblastoma multiforme tumors (WHO grade IV) are rapidly growing, hypercellular tumors with areas of necrosis and increased vascularization. Unfortunately, glioblastoma multiforme are the most common type of astroblastoma and carry the worst prognosis (Fig. 2.1) [3, 5].

Neuroepithelial Tumors (Gliomas)

Most gliomas arise from the functional tissue of the brain and are associated with swelling (edema) and sometimes bleeding (hemorrhage), which can also alter the structure and function of the normal brain. The location, growth rate, and growth pattern of the tumor determine its effects on brain function [3]. Mass effect, which is caused by the tumor compressing normal brain tissue, or brain infiltration by these tumors can cause depressive phenomenon (neurological deficits such as weakness and blindness) and irritative phenomenon (seizures). They can also occlude arteries or veins and cause strokes or interfere with the flow and absorption of cerebrospinal fluid (CSF), causing hydrocephalus. The most malignant variants of gliomas (glioblastoma multiforme) can create their own blood supply and steal blood from normal brain [3, 5].

Clinical Presentation

The most common symptoms of brain tumors are headache, seizures, and progressive neurological deficit. Headaches can be caused by increased intracranial pressure, invasion or

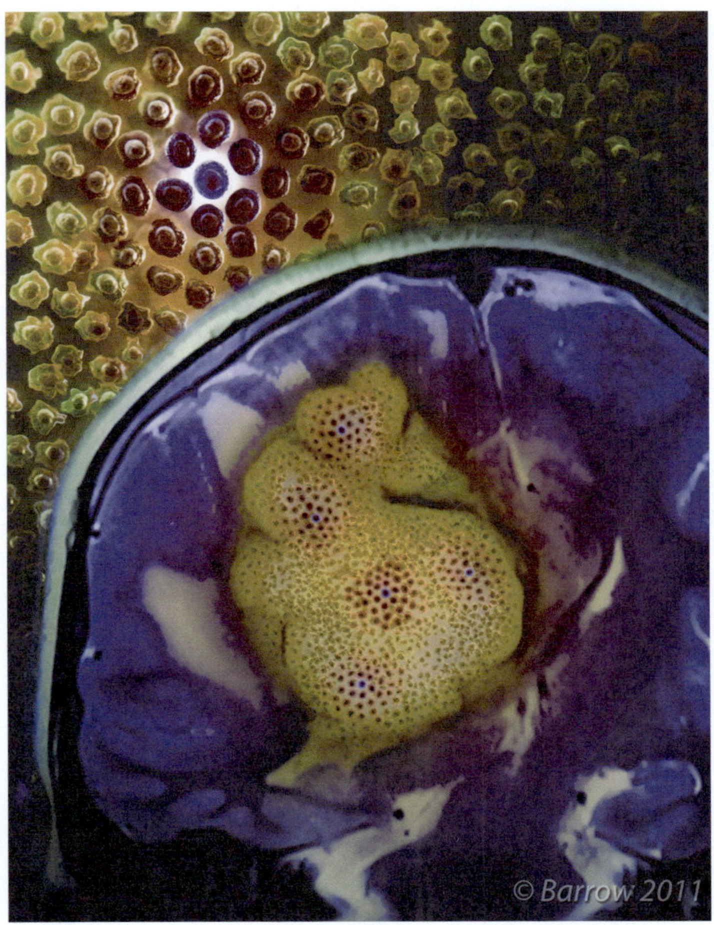

FIGURE 2.1 Artist's illustration of a large malignant brain tumor (*green area*) in the parietal region of the brain. The pressure over the normal brain is so severe that is shifting the brain from left to right (brain herniation). It is also infiltrating the surrounding brain tissue, causing severe swelling and brain dysfunction (Reprinted with permission from Barrow Neurological Institute)

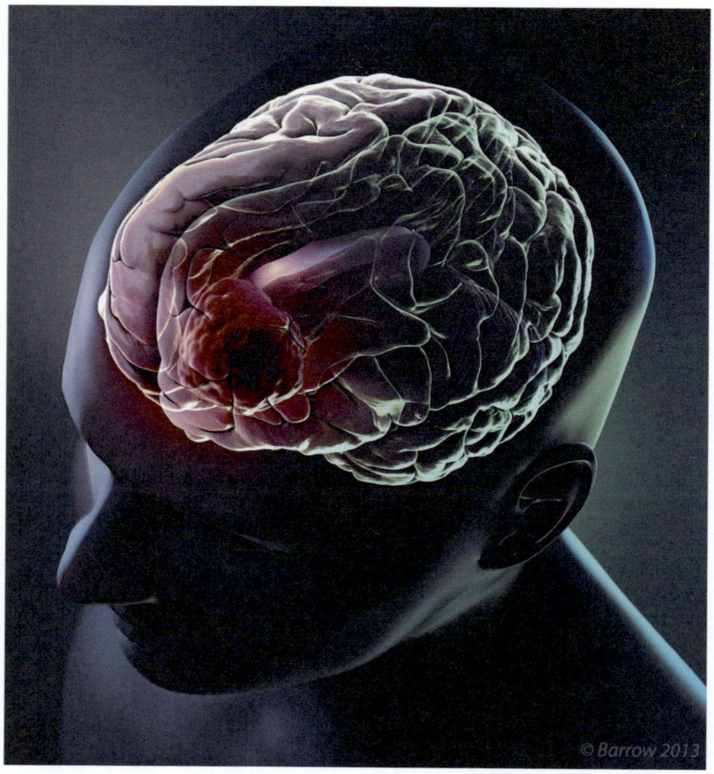

FIGURE 2.2 Artist's illustration of a malignant brain tumor (*red area*) located at the left frontal lobe, causing mass effect and brain herniation. Tumors in this locations can cause language problems (aphasia) and personality problems, memory alterations, and in cases of large tumors, weakness and sensation abnormalities over the right side of the body (Reprinted with permission from Barrow Neurological Institute)

compression of sensitive structures, and vision problems. Other worrisome symptoms include double vision with headaches, hearing loss with dizziness, and gradual onset of speech difficulty. Changes in behavior, memory loss, loss of concentration, and general confusion may all be subtle signs

(Fig. 2.2). Increased intracranial pressure due to large tumors frequently causes nausea, vomiting, dizziness, vertigo, and changes in mental status. Acute deterioration is not uncommon and is caused by tumor swelling (Fig. 2.2), hemorrhage, infarction, or hydrocephalus [3, 5].

Clinical Symptoms According to Location

Frontal Lobe Tumors can cause problems in cognition, behavior, speech, and movement. Patients lose their energy for intellectual, physical, and social activity. They are also impulsive, lose social inhibition, and have fluctuating emotions. Motor aphasia (difficulty speaking) and agraphia (difficulty writing) may also be present (Fig. 2.2).

Temporal Lobe Tumors cause alterations in hearing, language, vision, behavior, and movement. Sounds are heard but not appropriately interpreted. Tumors in this location may cause auditory illusions or hallucinations. Patients sometimes have difficulty understanding spoken language.

Parietal Lobe Tumors produce sensory problems. Other symptoms are difficulty dressing oneself, denial of extremity weakness, lack of awareness of objects, and constructional apraxia, which is the inability to build or draw objects. Failure to recognize familiar faces is also common.

Occipital Lobe Tumors cause vision problems, including blindness in one or both eyes, visual hallucinations and illusions, and abnormal or multiple images of a single object.

Diagnosis

The diagnosis of a brain tumor is based on a combination of the patient's clinical symptoms and a neurological examination performed by a neurologist or a neurosurgeon. In addition, a diagnostic imaging test is always necessary, usually either computed tomography (CT) or magnetic resonance imaging (MRI) are used. MRI not only confirms the diagnosis but also gives valuable information regarding the characteristics, size, and location of the tumor [1].

After diagnostic imaging has demonstrated the presence of a brain tumor, the most accurate method for identifying the type of tumor is with a biopsy. A biopsy is a surgical procedure in which a sample of the brain tumor is removed and is then examined under the by a pathologist. Biopsy results confirming the final diagnosis usually take 4–7 days.

Treatment

Treatment of a malignant brain tumor is complex and requires the efforts of a multidisciplinary team of specialists. The team consists of a neuro-oncologist, neurosurgeon, neuropathologist, neurologist, oncologist, radiation oncologist, physical therapist, occupational therapist, and speech pathologist. The role of the neurosurgeon includes biopsy of the tumor for the purpose of diagnosis, reduction of the tumor mass to the greatest extent possible with preservation of neurological function, and application of adjuvant therapies on the basis of clinical and laboratory observation [4].

Medical Therapy

In general, all patients with malignant brain tumors, regardless of whether they undergo a neurosurgical procedure, should be prescribed a course of steroids after the diagnosis has been confirmed on an MRI. Steroids decrease brain swelling caused by the brain tumor, sometimes they also diminish the mass effect and improve the clinical symptoms. Usually, the preferred steroid for a malignant brain tumor is dexamethasone. Depending on the location, brain tumors can cause seizures, and for that reason patients should be on prophylactic antiepileptic drugs.

Surgery

The role of surgery is to obtain a biopsy specimen and to remove the tumor mass. Patients with malignant brain tumors commonly undergo multiple surgeries in order to control tumor recurrence. Oncological control is achieved with tumor removal, which usually delays recurrence and enhances adjuvant therapy. Unfortunately, surgery does not completely cure a malignant brain tumor. Sometimes total removal of the tumor is not possible because of the location or diffuse tumor infiltration into brain tissue; however, partial resection may still provide an advantage compared with a biopsy alone [4].

Complications and Risk of the Surgery

Patients undergoing surgical procedures should be aware of the complications and risks and should have a clear understanding of the goals of the surgery. Potential complications may include pain, infection, bleeding, cerebrospinal fluid leak, blindness, deafness, stroke, paralysis, language problems, coma, and even death.

Postoperative Phase

After surgery, patients are admitted to the neurointensive care unit where they stay for 48–72 h. Usually, they are extubated and awake; however, sometimes the surgeon and the anesthesiologist will decide to keep the patient sedated and intubated. Patients will have pain at the incision site, will be nauseous and may experience vomiting, and will be mildly confused for few hours. These symptoms are usually related to the anesthesia. If possible, patients should get out of bed and walk within 24 h after surgery. Doing so helps prevent deep venous thrombosis (blood clots) in the legs. Patients are maintained on steroids and antiepileptic drugs for a while after surgery. An MRI is usually performed within 24–48 h to evaluate postoperative inflammatory changes and residual tumor. Restrictions on diet and activity are gradually lifted, but patients should be back to a full diet and should be walking within 48–72 h after surgery [5].

Adjuvant Therapy

Adjuvant therapies are therapies used to forestall or treat recurrences. Radiation therapy and chemotherapy are the principal types of adjuvant therapy for patients with malignant brain tumors [1, 2].

Radiation therapy is started within days after surgery and after the diagnosis of malignant brain tumor has been histologically confirmed and is continued for 2 or 3 weeks. Side effects from radiation therapy include nausea, vomiting, generalized weakness, and hair loss. Complications can include brain edema (swelling), demyelination (loss of myelin, a substance that helps preserve the integrity of nerve signals), and necrosis. Demyelination is usually self-limited and does not require treatment. Radiation necrosis occurs 4–40 months after radiation; when present, it is progressive and irreversible [2].

Recent advances in chemotherapy have led to drugs with fewer side effects and better tumor control. There are two types of chemotherapy drugs: drugs that kill cancer cells (cytotoxic) and drugs that prevent cells from reproducing (cytostatic). Temozolomide is one of the most commonly used drugs. It is an oral drug that kills malignant cells and enhances the response of malignant gliomas to radiation. It has a low toxicity profile with good penetration into the brain. Other chemotherapy drugs include nitrosoureas, platinums, procarbazine, vincristine, irinotecan and etoposide. The common side effects include: nausea, vomiting, loss of hair, diarrhea, constipation, neuropathy, low platelets, low white cells, and anemia [5].

Prognosis

Factors that can affect a patient's length of survival include age, overall quality of life, tumor size and location, and even marital status. Unfortunately, the prognosis for patients with malignant brain tumors (high-grade glioma) is poor. The median survival is less than 2 years. For patients with anaplastic glioma (WHO Grade III) the median survive is 2–5 years. Only a small number of patients with high-grade gliomas have lived longer than 2 years. After extensive surgery and treatment, recurrence is inevitable, and patients will eventually succumb to this disease [3, 5].

References

1. Binello E, Green S, Germano IM. Radiosurgery for high-grade glioma. Surg Neurol Int. 2012;3:S118–26.
2. Bradley D, Rees J. Updates in the management of high-grade glioma. J Neurol. 2014;261(4):651–4.
3. Greenberg MS. Handbook of neurosurgery. New York: Thieme; 2010.
4. Hart MG, Garside R, Rogers G, Stein K, Grant R. Temozolomide for high grade glioma. Cochrane Database Syst Rev. 2013;(4), CD007415.
5. Quinones-Hinojosa A. Malignant gliomas: anaplastic astrocytoma, glioblastoma multiforme, gliosarcoma. In: Winn HR, editor. Youman's neurological surgery. Philadelphia: Elsevier; 2011.

Chapter 3
Pituitary Tumors

David S. Baskin

The Pituitary Gland

The pituitary gland is a small organ about the size of an acorn located at the base of the brain. It is surrounded by a bony saddle-like structure above the sinuses at the back of the nose, called the sella turcica. The pituitary gland is sometimes referred to as the "master gland of the body" because it releases substances which control the basic functions of growth, metabolism, and reproduction.

The pituitary gland is divided into two parts called lobes. Each lobe releases special substances, or hormones, which control basic activities within the body. The many influences of the pituitary gland on body systems is seen in Fig. 3.1, and listed in Table 3.1.

Understanding Your Symptoms

A tumor in the pituitary gland causes symptoms by either releasing too much of a hormone or by pressing on the gland causing it to release too little hormone. The symptoms one

D.S. Baskin, MD, FAANS
Department of Neurosurgery,
Houston Methodist Hospital, Houston, TX, USA
e-mail: dbaskin@tmhs.org

A. Agrawal, G. Britz (eds.), *Emergency Approaches to Neurosurgical Conditions*, DOI 10.1007/978-3-319-10693-9_3,
© Springer International Publishing Switzerland 2015

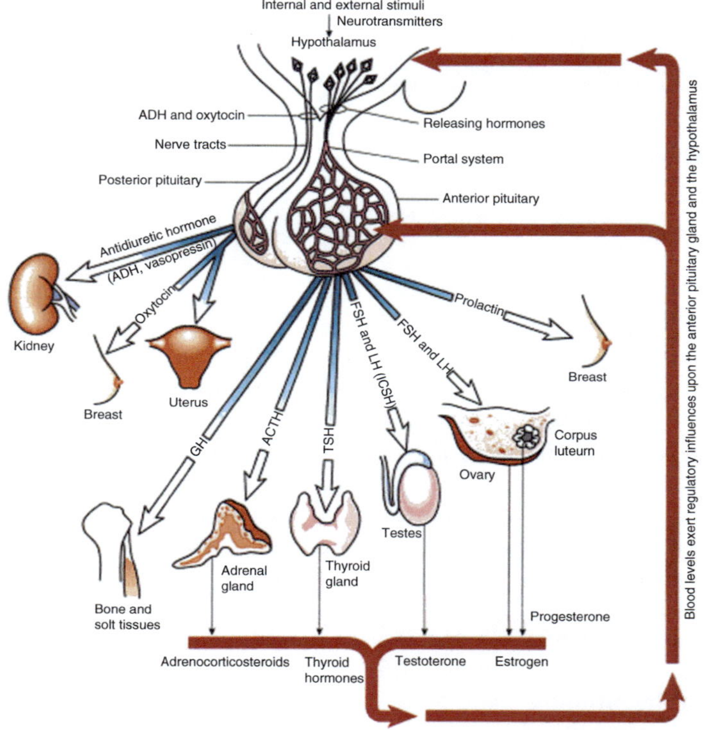

FIGURE 3.1 The pituitary gland and it effect and regulation of other body tissues. The pituitary gland is responsible for regulating many body tissues. Breast function in females, steroid production by adrenal glands, thyroid function, bone growth and health, sexual function in men and women, fluid and electrolyte and water balance, and contraction of the uterus during childbirth are just some of the functions that it regulates. There is a complex balance of feedback loops between the various body organs and the pituitary that enables the body to function optimally

experiences from the pituitary tumor are determined by the type of tumor. A pituitary tumor may also cause symptoms by growing and pressing on the structures surrounding the pituitary gland, like the nerves to the eyes.

TABLE 3.1 Pituitary hormones and their functions and effects on the body

Anterior lobe	Function
Thyroid stimulating hormone (TSH)	Causes the thyroid gland to grow and release thyroid hormones (called T4 and T3)
Adrenocorticotropic hormone (ACTH)	Causes adrenal gland to release several hormones. The major one is cortisol. Several others are also released
Growth hormones (GH)	The main hormone for general body growth. Growth hormone regulates many metabolic functions including how the body handles glucose
Follicle stimulating hormone (FSH)	Stimulates ovulation in women and the production of sperm in men.
Luteinizing hormone (LH)	Stimulates ovulation in women and testosterone production in men.
Prolactin (PRL)	Causes breast enlargement and breast milk. Too much causes infertility in women and impotence in men
Posterior lobe	**Function**
Antidiuretic hormone (ADH)	Controls thirst and the amount fluid reabsorbed into the bloodstream and the amount of urine produced by the kidneys.
Oxytocin	Stimulates uterine contractions in women. Its function in men is unknown, if any.

This chart summarizes the effects of the hormone of the pituitary gland on various bodily functions. Each hormone has a number of very specialized effects, and this chart only summarizes these complicated hormonal interactions. There is a delicate cycle of secretion and regulation of these functions that varies by time of day and the degree to which a person is physically and psychologically stressed. Each of these hormones can be tested using a variety of different types of studies. They can be tested by simply measuring the individual hormone levels in the blood, but they can also be tested by stimulation or suppression tests that tell the doctors how well the body's balance and regulation of these hormones is working

A pituitary tumor can cause an increase in any of the anterior pituitary hormones listed in Table 3.1. For example, you may experience the following:

In a condition called acromegaly [1, 2], an increase in the amount of growth hormone (GH), causes the body to grow at an abnormally fast rate. Bones become thicker and the hands and feet may appear wider or bigger, and the jaw may protrude. Carpal tunnel syndrome and spinal problems may develop due to excessive growth of bone and soft tissue. Many patients develop diabetes, high blood pressure, and cardiac problems. This tumor shortens life span.

In Cushing's disease [2, 3], a tumor releases adrenocorticotropic hormone (ACTH) which produces an increase in the body's own steroid called cortisol, which leads to fat deposits, especially in the shoulders and face, and increased growth of body hair. Brittle diabetes and severe high blood pressure that can be difficult to control, even with many medications, is common. Patients often develop softening of the bones, called osteoporosis. Left untreated, this is a life threatening problem.

With a tumor making too much prolactin called a prolactinoma [2, 4, 5], elevated levels of prolactin may cause secretion of breast fluids and decreased sexual drive and breast enlargement in men and women. It may also cause irregular or absent menstrual periods in women, and difficulty in having an erection or infertility in men. Many women note weight gain and mood swings. Men may have a decrease in testosterone levels because of this tumor.

For pituitary tumors that do not secrete hormones [2], the initial symptoms may not occur until the tumor presses on the structures surrounding the normal pituitary gland. This is why such tumors are often quite large when they are discovered.

Because the pituitary gland is located near the eyes, it can press on the nerves to the eyes and cause loss of vision. Loss of peripheral vision (See Fig. 3.2) may occur first and be undetected. This may progress to eventual blindness if the pressure is not removed from the nerves. Almost any

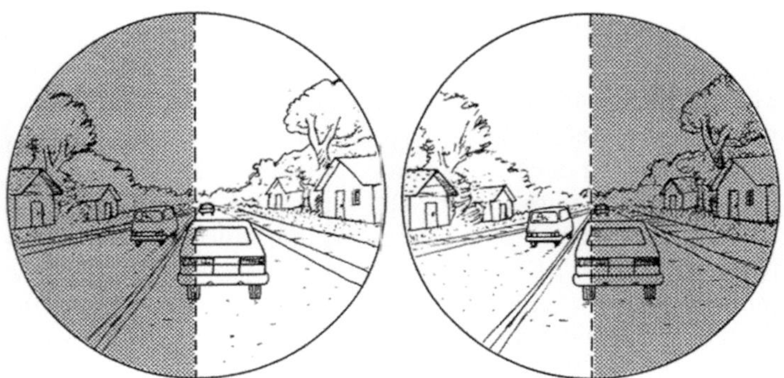

FIGURE 3.2 Visual problems from pituitary tumors. There are many different types of visual problems that can occur when a pituitary tumor grows upwards and presses on the optic nerves or their connections. The most common problem is to lose vision in the outer fields, called a bitemporal hemianopsia. Often patients do not notice this, as they correct for the problem by moving their head back and forth. Doctors perform an examination called a visual field test in order to detect what quadrants of vision may not be functioning correctly

kind of visual problem can be seen with large pituitary tumors. The tumor may also press on the nerves that move the eye and cause double vision. If the tumor is very large it may press on other parts of the brain and cause problems with memory, weakness, numbness, or increased pressure in the brain because of impaired circulation of the brain fluid.

Treatment Options

Most pituitary tumors can be cured or at least very well controlled with the treatments that are available. Treatment options include observation over a period of time to see if treatment is needed, treatment with drugs, radiation therapy, and surgery

Observation Without Treatment

Since most pituitary tumors are usually benign, some tumors may be observed without treatment because they may grow very slowly. If a decision is made to observe the tumor, ongoing evaluations with CT or MRI scans, and assessment by an endocrinologist and possibly an ophthalmologist will be performed. CT or MRI scans will be performed within 3–6 months after the initial diagnosis and every 6–12 months thereafter until the situation has been clarified. This period of observation without treatment provides information that helps the doctors decide whether other treatments that have more risks are needed.

Observation without treatment may also be recommended if conditions are present that would seriously increase the risk of surgical or other treatments. Because pituitary tumors are slow growing, patients can often be observed without treatment for long periods of time without the tumor causing serious problems. This can be the recommended form of treatment for patients who are age 70 or above or who have a serious medical illness such as heart disease. Close follow-up will be necessary to monitor tumor growth and symptoms.

Treatment with Drugs

Only one type of pituitary tumor can be successfully treated with drugs. This type of tumor, called a prolactinoma, secretes a hormone called prolactin.

Prolactinomas can often by controlled by a drug called Bromocriptine, or another newer drug called Cabergoline [5]. These drugs will often reduce the size of the tumor and at the same time produce a decrease in the abnormally high prolactin level in the blood. Although the drugs may control the tumor, they will not cure it. Treatment in most cases must be continued for many years. While these drugs are effective in many cases, some patients develop nausea, headache, dizziness, and weakness while taking them. Usually these symptoms can be reduced by taking small doses of the drug at first and slowly increasing the dosage up to the needed level over a period of several weeks or months. These drugs will not control all prolactin-secreting tumors. For approximately 20 % of patients with prolactinomas, surgery or radiation therapy may be needed.

Focused Radiation Therapy/Stereotactic Radiosurgery

Another treatment option for pituitary tumors is radiation therapy. Radiation therapy is most commonly used after surgery. Most people think of radiation therapy as a treatment for malignant tumors. As previously mentioned, most pituitary tumors are benign and not malignant. Even though most pituitary tumors are benign, some tumors have roots in the bone or coverings around the brain that involve vital nerves or blood vessels in such a way that surgical removal would cause significant damage to these important structures. In these cases it is best to treat the main part of the tumor with surgery and to use radiation therapy for the roots or remaining tissue.

Radiation therapy, given under the direction of specialist called a radiation oncologist, is most effective when the size of the tumor has been reduced by surgery. The greater the amount of tumor at the time of radiation therapy, the less effective the treatment will be.

A specialized form of radiation therapy called "stereotactic radiosurgery" can be used in most cases. Radiosurgery involves a highly focused radiation treatment. The patient can often return home after a single treatment, which is done as an outpatient. There are minimal to no side effect with this type of treatment.

Surgery

Surgery is the preferred method of treatment for most pituitary tumors. Two types of operations are done for the removal of pituitary tumors. One, called a craniotomy, is directed through the skull above the eye. The other, called a transsphenoidal operation, is directed through the nose. The craniotomy operation involves making an incision on the scalp near the top of the head. A piece of bone is then lifted out and the coverings over the brain are opened. The lower part of the brain is gently lifted to expose and remove the tumor. The piece of bone is then replaced and the scalp is closed with stitches or staples. In most cases, the incision on the head can be placed so that the hair hides the scar. This type of operation is usually not needed for a pituitary tumor, but it is sometimes necessary if the tumor is very large and/or it cannot be reached through the nose by a transsphenoidal operation.

The transsphenoidal operation is the most common operation for a pituitary tumor [6] (Fig. 3.3). The surgical approach for this operation is through the nose. There is no incision on the face. This surgical approach provides the best exposure of the tumor at the lowest risk. The operation normally takes 2 or 3 h. Following the operation, most patients spend one day in the intensive care unit before returning to their hospital room. Patients usually stay in the hospital for 1 or 2 days following the operation. In some cases, patients are sent home the day after surgery. The best form of transsphenoidal surgery today is called endoscopic endonasal surgery [6] (see Fig. 3.4)

Risks of Surgery

Certain risks exist with both the craniotomy and the transsphenoidal operation. With either operation there is a small risk to life (less than 1 %) as occurs with any anesthesia and major surgery. With either operation there is a risk to developing problems with vision because the nerves to the eyes are located in the area of the tumor. When there has been a distinct loss of vision before the operation due to pressure from the tumor, vision is often greatly improved by the operation. The degree of recovery of vision after the operation depends on how much damage has been done to the nerves of the eye by the tumor before the operation.

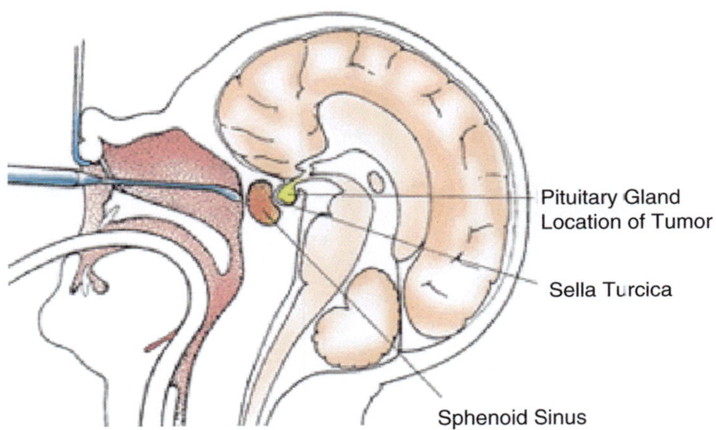

FIGURE 3.3 The transsphenoidal approach to the pituitary gland. This surgical approach takes advantage of the fact that the pituitary gland is located on top of a hollow air sinus at the base of the skull. Using an approach through the nasal passages, one can enter into the sinus, remove the bone separating the sinus from the pituitary, and then remove the tumor without damaging any of the brain structures. Advances and technology have provided very high resolution pictures (1080 P or Blu-ray type definition) from the endoscopes that are now used to remove these tumors. The surgery has been converted into a very high-risk procedure with a prolonged recovery time to a minimally invasive operation with a very rapid return to work and minimal side effects

There is some risk that surgery may damage the pituitary gland. In many cases pressure by the tumor has already damaged the gland. The chance of surgery damaging the gland is small if the tumor is small, however the risk increases when the tumor is large. In most cases, even with very large tumors, the gland regains some function after a recovery period.

Another risk is a condition called Diabetes Insipidus, which is caused by a decrease in antidiuretic hormone (ADH). A lack of this hormone leads to increased thirst and frequent urination. Diabetes Insipidus can be treated by replacing the antidiuretic hormone with medication. This is

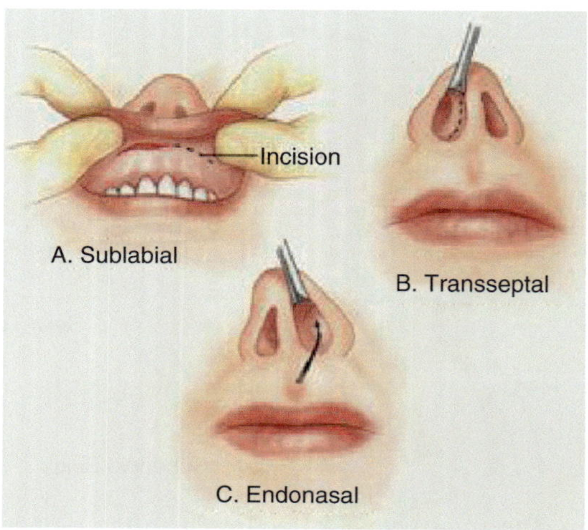

FIGURE 3.4 Modern day surgical approaches to the pituitary gland. In recent years, surgery to remove pituitary tumors has been primarily through the nasal passages, rather than using more invasive approaches in which the skull is opened. (**a**) The older and more classical approach is to remove pituitary tumors is via an incision underneath the lip, which provides access to the nasal passages. This procedure produces numbness in the teeth and requires a more extensive recovery, usually involving a prolonged period of sinusitis and the use of nasal packs and splints. (**b**) A more recent development is the use of the transseptal approach, where an incision was made in the front of the nose to gain access to the pituitary region. While this is an advance, it still involves an extensive nasal dissection and a more prolonged recovery because of symptoms and complications relating to manipulation of the nasal structures. (**c**) Using the endoscopic endonasal approach, there is no dissection through the nasal structures. The sinuses are entered into in the very back of the nose, with excellent exposure of the pituitary gland and its surrounding structures. This is the least invasive technology available for removal of pituitary tumors today, and provides optimal surgical exposure, the least number of nasal complications, and excellent outcomes

usually given in the evening to reduce the frequency of urination during the night. Diabetes insipidus resolves in a few days in most patients.

Other risks associated with surgical intervention include double vision, numbness of the face, bleeding, infection, stroke, or other neurological defects.

Transsphenoidal Operation

Most pituitary tumors are removed by the surgical procedure called a transsphenoidal operation (See Fig. 3.3). Transsphenoidal means the operation is directed through the sphenoid bone and sinus. The sphenoid is a small bone in the back of your nose located just below the pituitary gland. It often contains a large air filled cavity called the sphenoid sinus. In the past the transsphenoidal operation was begun by making a 1–2 in. incision under your lip at the top of your upper gum in the sublabial modification of the transsphenoidal approach (See Fig. 3.4a) or within the nose in the transseptal modification. (See Fig. 3.4b). In recent years the operation has been modified so that there is no need for an incision under the lip or in the front part of the nose in most patients. The new procedure is called an endonasal procedure because the tumor is approached through the nasal cavity without an incision under the lip or in the front part of the nose. There is no incision on the face. The tumor is reached by working through one nostril, and making a hole at the back of the nose (See Fig. 3.4c) into the sphenoid sinus and then exposing the pituitary gland. The tumor is then removed. The endonasal endoscopic procedure reduces the time required in the operating room by as much as 2 h. The newer approach has proven to be as effective as the older approach in reaching the pituitary gland, and the benefits are greater. Patients can resume a normal diet sooner after surgery, and the swelling of the face and risk of injury to the upper lip and teeth is markedly reduced. Post-operative discomfort is decreased and hospitalization has been shortened by as much as 2 days.

A small piece of fat is often removed from just below the skin on your abdomen to fill the cavity created by the tumor removal. The bottom of the skull is closed with a piece of bone or bone substitute. This will help to prevent leakage of cerebrospinal fluid (CSF), a fluid that surrounds the brain, spinal cord, and pituitary gland. At times a drain may be inserted into the spine while you are asleep to keep the pressure low and prevent leaking after surgery. The drain may also be used to push to tumor down by injecting fluid into it while you are under anesthesia.

In the endoscopic procedure, there is no need for stitches to close the area since no incision has been made in the nose or mouth. There is no need for gauze packing in the nose as is used when incisions have been made in the nose or mouth. There is minimal swelling, usually not noticeable.

Monitoring Your Fluid Balance

The pituitary gland secretes a hormone called antidiuretic hormone (ADH), which regulates the fluid in your body. After surgery, the amount of ADH circulating in the body may decrease. The decrease in ADH will cause the kidneys to release water from the body, producing large quantities of dilute urine. Also, the large loss of water from the body may produce dehydration, and therefore, more fluids will be needed. The deficiency of ADH is called Diabetes Insipidus. In most cases the deficiency resolves by the time you leave the hospital. The nursing and medical staff will be closely measuring both fluid intake and output. Therefore, it is important to keep an accurate count of everything you drink as well as your urine output.

Nasal Drainage

As mentioned previously under the description of the operation, a small piece of fat is removed from just under the skin over the abdomen to "plug" the opening in the back of your nose. The medical and nursing staff will also be monitoring the drainage from your nose. This is done by changing the pad covering your nose and monitoring the drainage for cerebrospinal fluid (CSF), which would indicate a leak. You will also have a small dressing on your abdomen where the "plug" of fat was removed. The stitches from this incision will dissolve by themselves and do not need to be removed. It is important to note that there is always some draining from the nose. You will be started on nasal decongestants and nasal saline the day after surgery. Continued use of these items for the first 30 days after surgery is recommended.

Pain After Surgery

Usually the pain after surgery is mild. You may experience a headache, which can be treated with medication. You may have some bruising under your eyes and/or along the side of your nose. This should resolve by itself within several weeks. Your nose will be stuffy, and you may have to breathe through your mouth for the first few days to weeks, as if you had a bad cold (Fig. 3.5).

Recovering from Your Surgery

In most patients the body will adapt to the changing levels of antidiuretic hormone (ADH) and maintain a reasonable balance of fluid. However, for a small number of patients urine production remains too high. If this occurs, your doctors may begin temporary treatment with an injection of synthetic ADH. If the body continues to be unable to control urine production, you may need to take the ADH hormone after you leave the hospital. If this occurs, you will probably be given a form of ADH, which can be taken as nose drops or spray, or a tablet.

During the weeks or months after surgery repeat hormone tests and eye exams are commonly needed. These tests will be

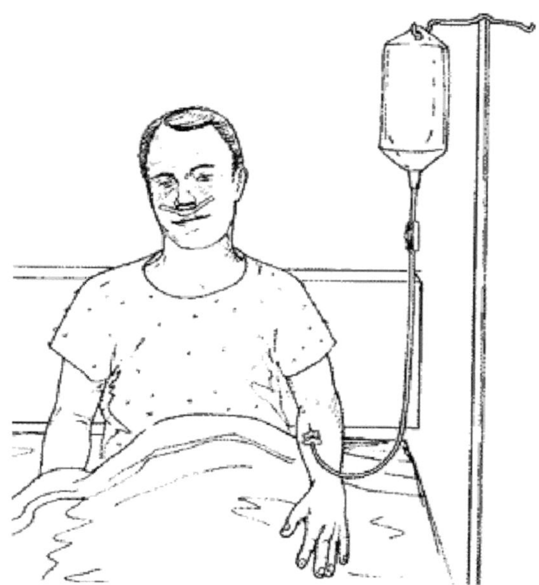

FIGURE 3.5 Fluid and electrolyte balance. After surgery, doctors will carefully monitor the amount of fluid going into your veins as well as your urine output. A flexible plastic catheter called an intravenous catheter or IV will be used to give you additional fluids. This is because the pituitary gland regulates water balance in the body through a hormone called antidiuretic hormone. This hormone balance can be temporarily disturbed, causing too high or too low levels of sodium and other important minerals in the blood. Carefully monitoring your fluid balance with periodic blood tests will enable the doctors to ensure that your recovery is smooth and that there are no problems with water balance

similar to the ones that were done before the surgery. Often the doctors in your community can do these tests. The endocrinologist will test how well the pituitary gland is functioning by checking hormone levels in the blood. If the levels are not high enough for everyday activities the doctor may prescribe hormone replacement therapy. The ophthalmologist will evaluate any changes in your vision after the surgery.

Frequently, after the pressure from the tumor is relieved, visual problems will improve.

Discharge Instructions

If your tumor is small you will probably not have to take any hormone replacement after you are discharged from the hospital. Patients with decreased pituitary gland function can still lead a normal life by taking medication each day to replace the normal hormones in the body. If your tumor is large you may be given a medication called Hydrocortisone. This medication helps to protect your body from the effects of stress. If you need hydrocortisone after discharge, you may be instructed to increase the dose if you are stressed by fever, infection, surgery, or other illness. Other medications that may be needed for decreased pituitary function are thyroid medications; estrogen or progesterone in the female; and testosterone in the male.

Follow-Up Care

A follow-up appointment will be scheduled. Laboratory tests may be done at that time to check the hormone levels in your blood and urine. Some patients develop a low sodium level in the blood during the first week or two after surgery because the pituitary gland over compensates by producing too much antidiuretic hormone (ADH). The excess ADH causes the body to retain fluid thus diluting the serum sodium to low levels. The treatment for this is fluid restriction and replacement of sodium either by salt tablets or intravenously. For that reason you may be asked to obtain several sodium or electrolyte levels after leaving the

The decision to use radiation therapy is usually made at the time of a MRI scan several months after surgery. In most cases, a follow up appointment will be scheduled 4–6 months after the first follow-up appointment done approximately 6 week after surgery. The MRI scan is usually repeated at this time. If there are any visual changes due to the tumor, you should also see the ophthalmologist for studies of the visual fields. Laboratory tests may be obtained at this time and your medications will be reviewed.

Most patients with a pituitary tumor resume normal activities after treatment. Vision often improves if it was affected, and fertility improves in a number of patients who were infertile. Most individuals benefit tremendously from surgery, and go on to live fruitful and productive lives, improved by removing the tumor and eliminating its negative effects.

References

1. Melmed S. Medical progress: acromegaly. N Engl J Med. 2006;355:2558–73.
2. Lake MG, Krook LS, Cruz SV. Pituitary adenomas: an overview. Am Fam Physician. 2013;5:319–27.
3. Newell-Price J. Diagnosis/differential diagnosis of Cushing's syndrome: a review of best practice. Best Pract Res Clin Endocrinol Metab. 2009;23 Suppl 1:S5–14.
4. Klibanski A. Clinical practice. Prolactinomas. N Engl J Med. 2010;362:1219–26.
5. Colao A, Savastano S. Medical treatment of prolactinomas. Nat Rev Endocrinol. 2011;7(5):267–78.
6. Rotenberg B, Tam S, Ryu WHA, Duggal N. Microscopic versus endoscopic pituitary surgery: a systematic review. Laryngoscope. 2010;120(7):1292–7.

Chapter 4
Pediatric Brain Tumors

Mihir Gupta and Gerald A. Grant

Background

How Common Are Brain Tumors in Children?

Brain tumors are the second most common kind of cancer in childhood, but are still quite rare. Less than 4,000 new cases of all brain and spinal cord tumors combined are diagnosed in the United States each year. Brain tumors are roughly equally distributed across childhood age groups, but slightly more common among children between ages 1–4 and 15–19 years old.

What Causes Brain Tumors? Can They Be Inherited?

There is no known cause for the vast majority of these pediatric brain tumors. They are generally not inherited

M. Gupta, BA
Department of Neurosurgery, School of Medicine,
Stanford University, Palo Alto, CA, USA
e-mail: gupta5@stanford.edu

G.A. Grant, MD, FACS (✉)
Department of Neurosurgery, Stanford University Medical Center/
Lucile Packard Children' Hospital, Standord, CA, USA
e-mail: ggrant2@stanford.edu

A. Agrawal, G. Britz (eds.), *Emergency Approaches to Neurosurgical Conditions*, DOI 10.1007/978-3-319-10693-9_4,
© Springer International Publishing Switzerland 2015

from parents, nor are they expected to appear in a sibling of an affected child. In rare instances, a genetic syndrome may run in the family and create higher risk for certain brain tumors.

Symptoms

While each individual will experience different symptoms, tumors often produce patterns of symptoms depending upon their location in the brain. This is because each part of the brain controls unique functions or parts of the body. Common symptoms of tumors in each major area are listed in Table 4.1. Symptoms may appear on the opposite side of the body than the tumor is located, because some parts of the brain control the opposite side of the body. Speech and language is most often on the left side of the brain.

Hydrocephalus: A Common Complication of Many Brain Tumors

Normally, the brain contains several areas of fluid called ventricles. Hydrocephalus occurs when a tumor blocks normal fluid drainage of the brain, causing the ventricles to become dilated. The buildup of fluid and pressure can damage the brain or cause symptoms including headache and visual changes. A temporary solution for hydrocephalus is to install an external ventricular drain (EVD) that drains fluid from the ventricles to outside the body. In some cases, the EVD may be removed after the plumbing is restored and the hydrocephalus resolves. If long-term drainage is required, the EVD may be converted to a device called a shunt that diverts ventricular fluid to safe locations inside the body. Sometimes an endoscopic third ventriculostomy may be performed to avoid a shunt.

TABLE 4.1 Common symptoms of tumors located in different areas of the brain

Tumor location	Definition	Common symptoms
Supratentorial	Upper part of the brain	Headache
		Seizure
		Paralysis (opposite side of body)
		Speech and language difficulty
		Personality or memory change
Posterior fossa	Lower part of the brain	Headache
		Nausea, vomiting
		Eye movement changes
		Gait, balance or coordination difficulty
Brainstem	'Highway' for all signals between the brain and the body	Facial weakness, visual changes
		Gait or coordination difficulty
		Weakness
		Headache

Diagnosing Brain Tumors

Several tests help doctors to diagnose brain tumors. A brain scan with a computerized tomography (CT) or magnetic resonance image (MRI) may help to establish tumor size and location, as well as complications like bleeding or hydrocephalus. Doctors may obtain a <u>biopsy</u>, meaning a small sample of the tumor to examine in the laboratory.

TABLE 4.2 Common categories and subtypes of pediatric brain tumors

Category	Common subtypes
Glioma	Astrocytoma
	Grade I: pilocytic
	Grade II: fibrillary
	Grade III: anaplastic
	Grade IV: glioblastoma
	Ependymoma (Grade II or III)
	Optic glioma
Embryonal	Medulloblastoma
	SHH ('Sonic Hedgehog')
	WNT
	Group 3
	Group 4
	PNET
Sellar region tumors	Pituitary adenoma
	Craniopharyngioma
Germ cell tumors and cysts	Germinoma
	Embryonal carcinoma

The laboratory examines tumors at the molecular level in order to diagnose the specific tumor subtype. Each subtype may require different treatment. A <u>lumbar puncture</u>, or 'spinal tap,' may reveal tumor cells in the fluid that surrounds the brain and spinal cord.

Common Types of Pediatric Brain Tumors

The most common tumor categories and subtypes are listed in Table 4.2, and described further below.

Gliomas

Gliomas are the most common brain tumors in childhood. They are made up of a type of cells called glia. Normally, glial cells provide support to neurons in the brain, but can form a tumor if they start multiplying excessively. There are several types of gliomas, each requiring different treatment:

- Astrocytomas: the most common type of glioma

    - Grade I: generally slow growing and benign. May be removed by surgery or in some cases radiation.
    - Grade II: may be removed surgically, but often require additional chemotherapy and radiation
    - Grades III and IV: generally removed surgically with additional chemotherapy and radiation

- Ependymomas: tumors that arise from glial cells that normally line the ventricles of the brain. Often slow growing and benign, but may be higher grade. Generally removed with surgery followed by radiation therapy, and in some cases additional chemotherapy.
- Optic gliomas: tumors that affect the optic nerve, which carries visual information from the eye. These tumors generally cannot be removed by surgery, and are instead treated with chemotherapy or radiation. In some cases, they may be associated with a genetic syndrome called Neurofibromatosis.

Embryonal Tumors

These tumors arise from cells that normally help to form the brain early on in development.

- Medulloblastoma: once thought to be a single type of tumor, but molecular studies showed there are at least four distinct subtypes based on molecular markers: SHH (or 'Sonic Hedgehog'), WNT, Group 3 and Group 4. Chemotherapy and surgery regimens will likely be tailored specifically for each subtype.
- Primitive Neuroectodermal Tumor (PNET): generally removed with surgery, followed by radiation and chemotherapy in many instances.

Sellar Region Tumors

These tumors arise in a region of the brain called the pituitary gland that contains important glands controlling the body's hormones. Long-term follow up may be required because of the possible impacts on growth, hormone levels and vision. Treatment generally involves a combination of surgery, radiation and/or chemotherapy.

Germ Cell Tumors and Cysts

This family of tumors includes several subtypes that must be distinguished by molecular tests in the laboratory; treatment is tailored specifically to each subtype. A combination of radiation and chemotherapy is used in many of these tumors, and in some cases surgery will also be undertaken.

Other

There are also several other types of brain tumors that are more rare than those outlined above. Your treatment team will be able to provide information on the type of tumor as well as the treatment plan.

The Treatment Process

Treatment Teams

Caring for patients with brain tumors is an integrative team effort between several different professionals working together:

- Neurosurgeons: perform surgery to remove a tumor, care for patients recovering from surgery, and follow up with patients after they leave the hospital.
- Neurooncologists: specialists in the medical treatment of pediatric brain tumors and who prescribe chemotherapy

and other medications, but do not perform surgery. Neurooncologists also follow up with patients long-term.

- Endocrinologists: doctors who specialize in treating hormone imbalances caused by certain brain tumors around the pituitary gland.
- Radiologists: doctors who specialize in the imaging of brain tumors.
- Radiation oncologists are doctors who help treat brain tumors with radiation.
- Pathologists: doctors who examine tumors under the microscope and with specialized molecular tests in order to make a diagnosis or gauge tumor severity.
- Psychiatrists: doctors who specialize in mental and emotional health for patients, siblings and family members.
- Nurses: care for patients who are in the hospital, and also follow up with them in the clinic or by phone afterwards.
- Case manager/social worker: helps address financial, school-related and other needs for patients and families.
- Child life specialist: supports developmental and emotional needs for children and siblings.
- Chaplain: provides spiritual guidance and counseling for patients and families.

Family Accommodations During Treatment

Hospital stays may last for several days. Many hospital systems will have resources available to provide families a place to stay during that time. The case manager or social worker on the team can work with families to arrange housing.

Surgery

Surgery may be required to remove some or all of a tumor, or to obtain a small sample for diagnostic purposes. In some cases, surgery is not required. In other cases, the need for surgery will be evaluated after a period of close observation.

Surgery can help to reduce symptoms, but does not always cure a tumor permanently. For some tumors, surgery will be supplemented with chemotherapy and/or radiation therapy.

Chemotherapy

Chemotherapy involves using medications that target cancer cells. Chemotherapy may be used alone, or alongside surgery or radiation therapy. Some chemotherapy medications are given through an IV into the bloodstream, while others are given orally. Most chemotherapy regimens include more than one medication, in order to target more cancer cells. Chemotherapy is given one or more times per week, over a period of several weeks; more than one cycle of medications may be required. Chemotherapy medications may have side effects including nausea, fatigue, muscle aches and hair loss. In some cases, there may be additional medications available to reduce these side effects.

Radiation Therapy

It is sometimes possible to use focused radiation such as x-rays or gamma rays to target tumor cells. Radiation may be given in small doses over a period of time, often alongside chemotherapy or surgery. Side effects of radiation therapy may include nausea, fatigue, hair loss and brain swelling.

Other Medications

Several additional medications may help with complications of brain tumors or the side effects of therapy. Tumors may cause swelling of the brain called edema, which can be reduced with steroid medications; these medications are gradually tapered off over a few days or weeks. Some tumors can also cause seizures, and anti-seizure medications may help to reduce this risk. Anti-nausea medications may reduce the nausea and vomiting side effects of chemotherapy or radiation.

After Treatment

After any form of treatment, it is important to keep monitoring symptoms over a period of months or years. Regular follow-up appointments may include repeating brain scans every 3–6 months in order to gauge whether a tumor has increased in size or spread elsewhere. Your doctor can also discuss what symptoms may indicate that a tumor has recurred after treatment.

Frequently Asked Questions

Are There Any Nutrition or Dietary Requirements for a Child with a Brain Tumor? Are Any Foods Proven to Prevent Tumor Growth?

During chemotherapy or radiation, doctors may suggest certain foods to lower side effects like nausea, diarrhea or constipation. However, these diets only help with treatment side effects; there is no current evidence that any particular food has an impact on tumor growth.

Do Brain Scans Contain Radiation?

MRI scans do not use any radiation. However, an MRI can require a child to lie still for up to an hour, which may require sedating medication. CT scans contain small doses of radiation; they are much quicker than an MRI and often do not require sedation. A CT scan is often required in emergencies, or to rule out bleeding or fluid buildup.

Can Children Continue to Attend School? Will Their Performance Be Affected?

Radiation or chemotherapy may require missing school. Tumors may have short- or long-term impacts on cognitive functioning, depending on the area of the brain they occupy.

Can Children Continue to Participate in Physical Education Class or Sports?

The timeline for returning to these activities varies greatly depending upon the kind of tumor and therapy. Following surgery, the healing process may take 3–6 months or more. Chemotherapy and radiation may also affect the ability to do physical activity.

Do Brain Tumors Have Psychiatric Consequences?

Receiving the diagnosis of a brain tumor can have psychiatric effects on children as well as siblings, parents and other family members. For this reason, counselors and child life specialists are very important members of treatment teams.

Where Can I Learn About Clinical Trials for New Therapies?

All federally approved clinical trials are listed on the website www.clinicaltrials.gov. Your treatment team may also know about ongoing trials.

Can I Get Copies of Test Results and Hospital Records?

Every hospital has a department of records that can provide patients and families with a copy of all medical documents.

Some hospitals may also have secure online systems that can be used to view test results or communicate with the treatment team. You may also be able to have digital copies of imaging results loaded onto a CD.

Glossary of Common Terms

Benign   A benign tumor ford not usually spread to other parts of the body or invade surrounding tissue, though it may still cause symptoms because of its size. <u>Malignant</u> tumors, however, can spread to other parts of the body, a process known as <u>metastasis</u>.

Biopsy   A small piece of tissue that can be examined in the laboratory to diagnose a tumor. This is different from <u>resection</u>, which is an attempt to remove some or all of a tumor.

CT scan ("cat scan")   A common way to acquire images of the brain. Another common way is the <u>MRI scan</u>. Sometimes a <u>PET scan</u> may be used.

Cranial nerves   These nerves start in the brainstem and control many facial movements and sensation. They may be affected by tumors in the brainstem region.

Cystic   A tumor that contains fluid inside it.

Edema   A tumor may make molecules that cause water to leak out from blood vessels into brain tissue. <u>Steroids</u> may be given and tapered off over a few days or weeks to reduce edema and prevent symptoms from arising.

Grade   A classification of how abnormal the cells of a tumor look under a microscope. Tumor <u>stage</u>, on the other hand, describes how large the tumor has become and how far it has spread to other parts of the body.

Hydrocephalus   Normal areas of brain fluid (called <u>ventricles</u>) become overloaded with fluid, because a tumor is blocking drainage. An <u>external ventricular drain (EVD)</u> or a <u>shunt</u> may be required for treatment.

Inpatient   Treatment that requires staying overnight in the hospital. <u>Outpatient</u> treatment requires visiting the hospital during the day, and then returning home.

Lumbar Puncture ("spinal tap")   A procedure to collect fluid surrounding the spinal cord in the lower back. The fluid can be analyzed in the laboratory. A lumbar puncture may also be used to deliver medications directly to the fluid around the brain and spinal cord.

Molecular Classification   Tumors can be grouped into subtypes based on their specific molecular 'machinery,' and how their cells are 'programmed' by DNA. Each molecular subtype may have a different prognosis or may require different treatment.

Pathology   Looking at tissue under a microscope in order to help make a diagnosis or determine the severity of a tumor.

Port   A surgically implanted device under the skin in the chest that helps deliver medication, including some kinds of chemotherapy, to the bloodstream. This allows doctors to give medication or collect blood samples without the need for repeated needle sticks.

Primary   The first tumor to appear. The primary tumor may also metastasize, or spread to other areas in the body.

Prognosis   A 'forecast' of how a disease or symptoms are expected to progress.

Remission   A decrease in tumor size or symptoms. Partial remission means some decrease in symptoms, while complete remission means all symptoms have gone away and the tumor can no longer be detected. However, even a tumor in complete remission may reappear; this is called recurrence.

Chapter 5
Congenital Neurosurgical Problems

Herbert Edgar Fuchs

Spina Bifida and Tethered Cord Syndrome

The most common spinal anomaly is spina bifida, which occurs in several different forms varying in severity. Myelomeningocele is the open form of spina bifida, where the developing neural tube fails to close early in pregnancy, resulting in a portion of the incompletely developed spinal cord exposed through a skin defect on the back. Urgent surgery shortly after birth restores tissue coverage to the spinal cord, but cannot restore neurologic function. These infants also frequently have associated hydrocephalus (fluid on the brain), and Arnold-Chiari malformations (see below), requiring ongoing neurosurgical evaluation and treatment. In addition, the failure of the lower portion of the spinal cord to close results in bowel and bladder incontinence and orthopedic deformities, requiring other pediatric subspecialists often in a multidisciplinary spina bifida clinic setting. Due to the severity and life-altering nature of these deficits, there has been considerable interest in fetal surgery for the repair of myelomeningoceles in the uterus. A multi-center randomized

H.E. Fuchs, MD, PhD, FAANS, FAAP
Department of Surgery, Duke University
Medical Center, Durham, NC, USA
e-mail: fuchs001@mc.duke.edu

A. Agrawal, G. Britz (eds.), *Emergency Approaches to Neurosurgical Conditions*, DOI 10.1007/978-3-319-10693-9_5,
© Springer International Publishing Switzerland 2015

trial (MOMS Trial) has shown encouraging results to this approach, although with significant risk to both mother and fetus.

Spina bifida occulta is a term that encompasses the closed forms of spina bifida, where the skin over the spine is closed, but a variety of malformations result in a tethered cord, in which the bottom portion of the spinal cord is attached to structures within the spinal canal or subcutaneous tissues. The simplest of these is the fatty filum terminale, in which the normal thin tail of the spinal cord is thicker and less elastic, allowing tension on the spinal cord as the child grows. A lipomyelomeningocele is a fatty mass, similar to a mushroom erupting from the bottom of the spinal cord, and blending into the normal fat beneath the skin. A lumbar dermal sinus tract is a dimple, which may indicate a tract extending, and attaching to the bottom of the spinal cord. A split cord malformation is a more complex malformation in which a spike of bone may between two halves of the spinal cord. All of these conditions may affect the function of the bottom portion of the spinal cord, causing pain, numbness, and weakness of the legs, as well as bowel and bladder incontinence. For this reason, these patients are also ideally followed in a multidisciplinary spina bifida clinic.

Hydrocephalus

Hydrocephalus, or fluid on the brain, may be associated with a variety of conditions, including bleeding following premature birth, infection, trauma, tumors, or from other congenital malformations, such as myelomeningocele, as discussed above. The infant head normally grows in response to the growing brain. As fluid accumulates in hydrocephalus, the head size increases more rapidly, and the head size is seen to rise above the normal growth curve. The infant's skull soft spot is fuller, and firm, from increased pressure inside the skull. The infant may be irritable, or lethargic. Vomiting may occur, and the eyes may be seen to be looking down (sunsetting sign). The evaluation of such infants may include imaging studies with ultrasound, computerized tomography (CT), or magnetic resonance imaging (MRI) scans. Hydrocephalus may be treated with a shunt, in which a tube is placed to drain fluid to the abdominal cavity or to the heart to avoid the buildup of pressure. Cases in which there is an obstruction to the flow of spinal fluid within the brain may be amenable to endoscopic treatment to bypass the obstruction, and avoid shunt placement. Recently, studies have shown a potential benefit of combining an endoscopic third ventriculostomy with choroid plexus (the tissue that makes spinal fluid within the fluid chambers of the brain) cauterization, in an effort to avoid lifelong shunting. These studies are based on work done by Dr. Ben Warf during his time in Africa, treating predominantly post-infection cases.

Chiari Malformations

Chiari malformations involve the inferior portion of the skull and upper portion of the spine, along with the brainstem, spinal cord, and cerebellum. In the Chiari 1 malformation, the cerebellar tonsils protrude through the hole at the base of the skull through which the brainstem exits. Since this portion of the skull and spine is shaped like a funnel, the herniation of the tonsils into the upper portion of the spine results in compression of the junction of the brainstem and spinal cord, and interference with the normal flow of spinal fluid across this region. Symptoms of Chiari 1 malformation include headache at the base of the skull, especially with coughing, sneezing, or straining, numbness or weakness in the hands, and difficulty swallowing. A syrinx, or fluid pocket, may develop in the upper portion of the spinal cord. Evaluation of patients with Chiari 1 malformation includes MRI scanning. A Chiari malformation may cause, or be caused by, hydrocephalus. The treatment of Chiari 1 malformation is surgical, most often involving decompression.

Chiari 2 (or Arnold-Chiari) malformation is seen in patients with myelomeningocele, and represents a more severe form than Chiari 1 malformation, involving even the upper portions of the brain and brainstem. Swallowing and breathing difficulties are commonly seen, and this condition may be life-threatening. Evaluation involves MRI scanning, as well as evaluation of shunt function, as a shunt malfunction may make Chiari symptoms worse. Surgery for Chiari 2 decompression involves decompressing the lower portion of the brainstem, which may lie well down in the neck.

Arachnoid Cysts

Arachnoid cysts are fluid filled balloons occurring within the arachnoid layer covering the brain. The normal arachnoid is one of three covering layers of the brain and spinal cord, and is the layer that encloses the spinal fluid spaces. An arachnoid cyst arises early in development, when a separate pocket containing fluid forms. This balloon may compress adjacent areas of the brain, or may not cause any significant issues. For larger cysts causing neurologic problems, surgery is indicated. Such surgery may range from shunting the cyst, to endoscopic approaches to communicate the cyst space to the normal spinal fluid spaces, or to open surgery for cyst removal.

Encephaloceles

Encephaloceles are congenital defects of the coverings of the brain including the skull, which allow herniation of portions of the brain anywhere between the nose and back of the head. There may or may not be skin coverage of the herniated brain. Hydrocephalus is associated more commonly with encephaloceles more at the back of the head. Treatment of an encephalocele is surgical, with the intent to repair the defects in the covering layers of the brain, including the skull.

Craniosynostosis

The normal infant skull is composed of multiple plates of bone. Where these plates come together, the joints are called sutures. Where multiple sutures come together, are the soft spots, the most well known of which is the anterior fontanelle, just above the forehead. The sutures are the sites of skull growth. When a suture closes too early, growth at this site is lost, and the remainder of the skull must grow disproportionally to allow enough room for the growing brain. This condition is called craniosynostosis, and closure of a suture results in characteristic alterations in head shape, which may be diagnosed visually or with x-ray or CT scans. Closure of a single suture is associated with an 8–10 % chance of increased pressure on the developing brain, due to lack of adequate skull growth. Several genetic syndromes are associated with closure of multiple cranial sutures, with more severe deformities, and much greater chances of increased pressure on the brain. The treatment of craniosynostosis is surgical. For older infants, complex reconstructions of major portions of the skull may be performed usually in conjunction with a craniofacial team involving pediatric plastic surgery and neurosurgery. For infants diagnosed prior to 3–6 months, less invasive operations are possible. Over the last decade, increased emphasis has been placed on the potential for endoscopic surgeries to utilize much smaller incisions, followed by the use of specialized molding helmets to modify the abnormal head shape, with very encouraging results.

For Further Information

Spina Bifida Association: www.spinabifidaassociation.org – excellent website with lots of information for patients and families, sponsor an annual meeting.
Hydrocephalus Association: www.hydroassoc.org – excellent website with lots of information for patients and families, local chapters, and national conference.

Chapter 6
Hydrocephalus

Anthony M. Avellino

Introduction

Hydrocephalus is the abnormal accumulation of cerebrospinal fluid (CSF) within the ventricles (i.e., the fluid filled cavities within the brain) and subarachnoid spaces (i.e., the fluid filled space around the brain). It is often associated with dilatation of the ventricular system and increased intracranial pressure (ICP; i.e., increased pressure within the brain). The incidence of pediatric hydrocephalus as an isolated congenital disorder is approximately 1/1,000 live births. Pediatric hydrocephalus is often associated with numerous other conditions, such as myelomeningocele, tumors and infections. Hydrocephalus is almost always a result of an interruption of CSF flow and is rarely because of increased CSF production. In this chapter, we will discuss the clinical features, diagnosis, and treatment of pediatric hydrocephalus.

A.M. Avellino, MD, MBA
Department of Neurological Surgery, University of Washington
School of Medicine, Seattle, WA 98104, USA
e-mail: anthony.m.avellino@osfhealthcare.org

A. Agrawal, G. Britz (eds.), *Emergency Approaches to Neurosurgical Conditions*, DOI 10.1007/978-3-319-10693-9_6,
© Springer International Publishing Switzerland 2015

Clinical Features

Signs and symptoms of progressive hydrocephalus depend on age. The following outlines the signs and symptoms of hydrocephalus in premature infants, full-term infants, and older children.

Premature Infants

Hydrocephalus in premature infants is predominantly caused by post-hemorrhagic hydrocephalus (PHH), which occurs due to malabsorption of the CSF within the brain. Infants with PHH may have no symptoms or may exhibit increasing spells of apnea and bradycardia. If ventriculomegaly progresses and ICP increases, the anterior fontanelle becomes convex, tense, and nonpulsatile; and the cranial sutures splay and the scalp veins distend (Table 6.1).

Full-Term Infants

The common causes of hydrocephalus in full-term infants include aqueductal stenosis, Dandy-Walker syndrome, arachnoid cysts, tumors, and cerebral malformations. Symptoms include irritability, vomiting, and drowsiness. Signs include macrocephaly, a convex and full anterior fontanelle, distended scalp veins, cranial suture splaying, frontal bossing, cracked pot sound on percussing over dilated ventricles (positive Macewen's sign), poor head control, and the "setting-sun" sign, in which the eyes are inferiorly deviated (Table 6.1).

Older Children

Hydrocephalus after infancy is usually secondary to trauma or tumors. The predominant symptom is usually a dull and steady headache, which typically occurs upon awakening. It may be associated with lethargy, and often improves after vomiting. The headaches slowly increase in frequency and

TABLE 6.1 Signs and symptoms of hydrocephalus in children

Premature infants	Full-term infants	Older children
Apnea	Irritability	Headache
Bradycardia (i.e., low heart rate)	Vomiting	Vomiting
Tense fontanelle	Drowsiness	Lethargy
Distended scalp veins	Macrocephaly	Diplopia
Globoid head shape	Distended scalp veins	Papilledema
Rapid head growth	Frontal bossing	Lateral rectus palsy
	Macewen's sign	Hyperreflexia/clonus
	Poor head control	
	Lateral rectus palsy	
	"Setting-sun" sign	

severity over days or weeks. Other common complaints include blurred or double vision, decreased school performance and behavioral disturbances (Table 6.1).

Diagnosis

Hydrocephalus can be diagnosed by cranial ultrasonography in infants with open scalp fontanelles, and by CT and MR imaging, which will demonstrate increased ventricular size, as well as the site of pathological obstruction if present (e.g., tumors that obstruct the ventricles and produce ventriculomegaly).

Treatment

The treatment of hydrocephalus can be divided into non-surgical approaches and surgical approaches, which in turn can be divided into non-shunting or ventricular shunting procedures. The goals of any successful management of hydrocephalus are: (1) optimal neurological outcome and (2) preservation of cosmesis. The radiographic finding of normal-sized ventricles should not be considered the goal of any therapeutic modality.

Non-surgical Options

There is no non-surgical medical treatment that definitively treats hydrocephalus effectively. Historically, acetazolamide and furosemide have been used to treat hydrocephalus. Although both agents can decrease CSF production for a few days, they do not significantly reduce ventriculomegaly, and can lead to potential side effects such as lethargy, poor feeding, tachypnea, diarrhea, and electrolyte imbalances. While acetazolamide has been used historically to treat premature infants with PHH, recent studies have shown it to be ineffective in avoidance of ventricular shunt placement and to be associated with increased neurological morbidity.

Surgical: Non-shunting Options

Whenever possible, the obstructing lesion that causes the hydrocephalus should be surgically removed. For example, the resection of a tumor that obstruct the ventricles often treats the secondary hydrocephalus. Unfortunately, in most cases of congenital hydrocephalus, the obstructive lesion is not amenable to surgical resection.

For CSF obstruction at or distal to the aqueduct (e.g., tectal plate tumors, acquired aqueductal stenosis, or posterior fossa tumors), a potential surgical treatment is the endoscopic third ventriculostomy. By surgically creating an opening at the floor of the third ventricle, CSF can be diverted without placing a ventricular shunt. Recent studies report a high success rate for endoscopic third ventriculostomies among pediatric patients with hydrocephalus secondary to aqueductal stenosis.

Table 6.2 Common indications for ventricular shunt placement

Congenital hydrocephalus
Persistent post-hemorrhagic hydrocephalus
Hydrocephalus associated with myelomeningocele
Hydrocephalus associated with Dandy-Walker cyst
Hydrocephalus associated with arachnoid cyst
Hydrocephalus associated with posterior fossa tumor

Surgical: Ventricular Shunts

The following outlines the components of a ventricular shunt, and the potential shunt complications. In addition, Table 6.2 lists some of the common indications for placement of a ventricular shunt.

Components

CSF shunts are silicone rubber tubes that divert CSF from the ventricles to other body cavities where normal physiologic processes can absorb the CSF. Shunts typically have three components: a proximal (ventricular) catheter, a one-way valve that permits CSF flow out of the ventricular system, and a distal catheter that diverts the CSF to its eventual destination (i.e., peritoneal, atrium or pleural space). The most common type of ventricular shunt in use today is the ventricular to peritoneal shunt (i.e., shunt tubing from the ventricles to the peritoneal cavity which is the potential space around the organs in the abdomen).

Valves come in a variety of different pressure and flow settings depending on the manufacturer. However, a recent advance in shunt valve technology has been the introduction of programmable valves, which allows one to adjust the opening pressure settings of the implanted shunt valve without the need to subject the child to an additional surgical procedure to change valves.

Shunt Complications

Shunt complications and failure remain a significant problem in treating hydrocephalus. The goal in treatment of hydrocephalus with a ventricular shunt is to decrease intracranial pressure and associated brain damage and simultaneously prevent complications associated with the ventricular shunting procedure. Shunt complications fall into three major categories: (1) mechanical failure of the device, (2) functional failure because of too much or too little flow of CSF, and (3) infection of the CSF or the shunt device. However, the two most common complications are infection and obstruction, which are further explained below.

Shunt Infection

Despite the numerous measures used to decrease the risk of infection, in general, approximately 1–15 % of all shunting procedures are complicated by infection. Approximately three-quarters of all shunt infections become evident within 1 month of placement. Nearly 90 % of all shunt infections are recognized within 1 year of the last shunt manipulation, as it is believed that most bacteria are introduced at the time of surgery.

The most effective and widely used treatment of a shunt infection is to remove the infected shunt hardware and place an external ventriculostomy drain (i.e., placement of a tube within the ventricles and connecting it to an external sterile collection bag outside one's body). The patient is then treated with the appropriate intravenous antibiotics based on culture and sensitivity results. When the infection is cleared, a new ventricular shunt system is implanted, and the external ventriculostomy is removed.

Shunt Obstruction

Shunt obstruction is another common complication. Shunt devices are to be viewed as mechanical devices that can become obstructed or malfunction anywhere in their course and anytime during their lifetime. The most common scenarios occur weeks, months, or years after insertion, when choroid plexus or debris has occluded the proximal ventricular catheter tip. Another common shunt malfunction scenario is the child who has obstructed his distal catheter or has outgrown his peritoneal catheter, and presents with an obstruction after the distal catheter tip has slipped out of the peritoneal cavity. In addition, shunt valves can malfunction, and shunt tubing can break, disconnect or dislodge from its previous location.

Common symptoms of shunt obstruction depend on the age of the child. A child with a shunt malfunction often presents with signs and symptoms of increased brain pressure. Infants with a shunt malfunction usually present with irritability, poor feeding, increased head circumference, and/or inappropriate sleepiness. Children with a shunt malfunction usually present with headache, irritability, lethargy, nausea, and/or vomiting. However, it is important to inquire if the signs and symptoms that the child is presenting with are the same as those during a shunt malfunction in the past. The child can present with waxing and waning symptoms, or can alternatively present with a progressively worsening picture that does not improve until the shunt is revised. A child complaining of pain with a clinical picture consistent with shunt obstruction should not be given narcotics because of possible respiratory depression or arrest.

When a shunt malfunction is suspected, head imaging studies should be obtained after a careful history and physical examination. A head CT/MRI and anteroposterior and lateral skull, chest, and abdominal x-rays, are obtained to evaluate for increased ventricular size and shunt hardware continuity, respectively. Children who are diagnosed with a shunt malfunction are taken promptly to the operating room for shunt revision.

Summary

Signs and symptoms of progressive hydrocephalus depend on age. Symptomatic ventricular shunt malfunction should be evaluated, recognized and treated promptly to avoid undue morbidity. Ventricular shunt infection currently occurs in 1–15 % of children who have shunts placed or revised, and the majority of infections are detected within the first 1–6 months after a shunt procedure. The prognosis of pediatric hydrocephalus is dependent primarily on the underlying brain morphology (i.e., a child with relatively normal brain organization has a better outcome than a child with abnormal morphology).

Suggested References

1. Avellino AM. Chapter 4. Hydrocephalus. In: Singer HS, Kossoff EH, Hartman AL, Crawford TO, editors. Treatment of pediatric neurologic disorders. Boca Raton: Taylor & Francis Group; 2005. p. 25–36 (Portions of this chapter were reprinted/republished with permission of Taylor & Francis Group LLC Books; permission conveyed through Copyright Clearance Center, Inc).
2. Albright AL. Chapter 6. Hydrocephalus in children. In: Rengachary SS, Wilkens RH, editors. Principles of neurosurgery. 1st ed. London: Wolfe Publishing; 1994. p. 6.1–6.23.

Chapter 7
Chiari Syndrome

Samuel Braydon Harris and Richard G. Ellenbogen

Chiari I Malformation and Syringomyelia

Chiari I malformation (CMI) is a congenital or acquired malformation of the back of the brain. It involves the parts of the brain called the cerebellum, brainstem and the upper spinal cord. The cerebellum is a part of the brain that helps coordinate movement and balance. The brainstem is the main pathway for all signals from the brain to the spinal cord. There is no cognitive or "thinking" function associated with the cerebellum or brainstem, so patients with CMI can have normal cognitive function. A CMI is characterized by descent or "escape" of the cerebellum into the spinal canal through an opening at the base of the skull called the foramen magnum. Normally, the cerebellum is fully contained within the skull; however, in a CMI, a part of the cerebellum called the cerebellar tonsils, can be forced downward or escape into the

S.B. Harris
Columbia University,
116th St and Broadway,
New York, NY 10027, USA

R.G. Ellenbogen, MD, FACS (✉)
Department of Neurological Surgery,
University of Washington Medicine,
325 Ninth Ave, Seattle, WA 98104, USA
e-mail: rge@uw.edu

A. Agrawal, G. Britz (eds.), *Emergency Approaches to Neurosurgical Conditions*, DOI 10.1007/978-3-319-10693-9_7,
© Springer International Publishing Switzerland 2015

spinal canal and crowd the spinal cord and brainstem. This part of the cerebellum, the tonsils, can block the normal flow of fluid called cerebrospinal fluid (CSF) around the brain. At the same time the tonsils can compress the cervical spinal cord and brainstem, which are essential for normal brain function.

Chiari II malformation is associated with the birth defects, spina bifida (myelomeningocele) and hydrocephalus. Chiari II malformation (CMII) involves descent the middle structure of the cerebellum, the vermis, with descent of the brainstem below the foramen magnum. Chiari type III (and IV) malformations are severe and exceedingly rare varieties of the Chiari malformation. Only the more common CMI malformation will be discussed in this chapter, as its treatment is much different than the treatment for the other Chiari malformations.

The cause of the CMI brain malformation is unknown and is discovered in a wide range of ages from under 3 years of age to those over 60 years of age. The increased availability of MRI has increased the diagnosis of this condition, which was once thought to be rare. CMI is not as rare as once thought. If the cerebellum escapes more than 5 mm below the foramen magnum and the patient has typical clinical symptoms, than the patient may fit the diagnostic criteria for CMI. The exact incidence of the malformation is unknown, but in one hospital based study perhaps, 1/1,280 people or more had CMI based on MRI. We still do not know whether or not any person affected with CMI will pass it to their child. Although some cases have a genetic basis with more than on family member affected with CMI, this occurrence is quite rare. Thus siblings of CMI patients do not need an MRI unless they are suffering the same symptoms of CMI.

A simplified way of explaining the CMI to young patients is to describe it as a "size 10 brain stuck in a size 9 skull, " even though most of the patients do not suffer from a misshapen or small skull. There are two main pathological or abnormal events that are observed in each patient who has a CMI. There is 1) "escape" or herniation of the cerebellar tonsils into the spinal canal more than 5 mm and 2) blockage in the flow or circulation of CSF around the cerebellum. The herniation of the cerebellar tonsils through the foramen magnum can cause further problems by pushing on the spinal cord and brainstem. Normally, CSF pulses throughout the cranial vault and around the spinal canal in rhythm with the heartbeat of the patient. The altered CSF flow seen in patients with a CMI can result in some patients (from 10 to 60 %) developing a fluid collection within the spinal cord known as syringomyelia [1]. Syringomyelia is a cyst (syrinx) in the spinal cord that contains CSF that is trapped in the spinal cord (Photo I). A syrinx can expand the cord and cause damage to the normal nerve units as more CSF gets trapped. There are many theories of why this happens in some patients, but it does not happen in everyone. Syringomyelia, though not found in all patients with CMI, can lead to yet further neurological issues such as progressive motor, sensory and sphincter deficits and should be treated.

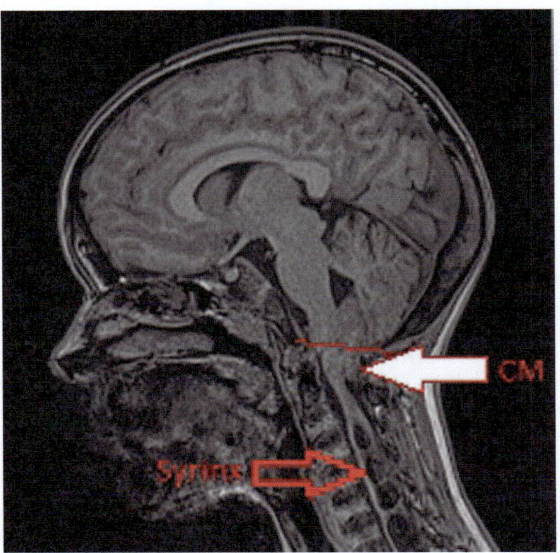

Table 7.1 Symptoms related to chiari I malformation

Headaches, "tussive": precipitated by coughing, straining, sneezing, etc.
General malaise, fatigue
Dizziness or "room spinning"
Eye symptoms- "to and fro" jerky movement, nystagmus
Change in gait or walking, balance issues
Swallowing problems
Sleep disturbances

Common Symptoms of CMI and Syringomyelia

CMI may cause specific symptoms related to CMI, and generalized symptoms that are often hard to associate only with CMI. Headaches and or neck pain, particularly precipitated by and exacerbated by coughing, straining, sneezing, are a very classic, specific symptom of CMI [2]. These headaches are called "tussive" headaches and can easily be distinguished from migraine headaches, which are unilateral and aggravated by light or noise. Frontal headaches occur in people without CMI and headaches associated with stress are not usual the result of this condition. Millions of Americans get headaches more than once a month, so physicians are cautious to avoid over diagnosing CMI based on headache symptoms that are not specifically tussive or in a person whose MRI that is not diagnostic for CMI but suffers headaches. Another less common symptom is a problem with balance and coordination, which may affect walking or other activities (See Table 7.1). CMI patients may complain about dizziness or vertigo (the room is spinning). Eye symptoms, most commonly jerky to-and-fro movements of the eyes, called nystagmus can be a complaint of CMI patients or be discovered on exam. CMI patients may complain about swallowing issues, sleep disturbances and general malaise in which they feel fatigued all the time. Some of that fatigue may be attributed from the incessant pain associated with headaches that start whenever the patient strains. It is important to note that a significant percentage of people with CMI suffer no symptoms and are diagnosed following an MRI for an unrelated clinical reason. These patients may remain asymptomatic for much of their life and the "natural history" (i.e., do they get symptoms later) of patients who do not receive treatment is still being studied.

Patients with syringomyelia associated with CMI can have severe symptoms, which include motor, sensory, pain and major dysfunction of their nervous system (See Table 7.2). The motor symptoms range from mild weakness to wasting of muscles. It is common for children with syringomyelia to have scoliosis as well. Syringomyelia can cause loss of feeling in the hands and feet or even the opposite. Patients can suffer exaggerated, hypersensitivity to touch, which is painful. The pain quality may be burning and occur in the arms and trunk. There may be joint pain in the shoulders that occurs from slow destruction of the joint. The major dysfunction of the nervous system may include incontinence of the bladder or bowel. There may be "autonomic" symptoms, which include wide swings in blood pressure, fainting or sweating. CMI patients with associated syringomyelia are rarely asymptomatic but their natural history is often one of progressively worse symptoms slowly over time.

Diagnosis

Magnetic Resonance Imaging (MRI) diagnosis of CMI sets the threshold for diagnosis by measuring the amount the cerebellar tonsils escape below the foramen magnum. Descent of 5 mm or greater is consistent with CMI. The MRI uses the interaction between strong magnetic fields produced by the machine and molecules in the body to produce high definition images of the body's internal structure. The advantage to using this technique is that in addition to the high resolution

Table 7.2 Neurologic signs in syringomyelia associated with chiari malformation [3]

Motor	Sensory	Pain	Sphincter	Autonomic
Weakness of hands and upper extremities	Decreased feeling in hands and arms	Midline pain	Urinary incontinence	Wide swings in blood pressure
Atrophy of hands or arms	Decreased sensation in torso	Burning pain in arms and torso	Bowel incontinence	Syncope of fainting
Increased tone or upper and lower extremities	Hypersensitivity to touch	Joint pain	Male impotence	Profuse sweating
Scoliosis	Decreased position sense	Joint pain	Bladder spasticity	Dysreflexia

of the brain and spinal cord it provides, it does not require the use of X-ray radiation that in large or cumulative doses can cause harm. To this date we do not have scientific proof that MRI can cause damage to the brain or spinal cord.

An MRI of the brain and spinal cord will be ordered if a CMI and syringomyelia are suspected based on symptoms. Some centers will add a CSF flow study in which the MRI evaluates the flow of CSF above and below the foramen magnum. A "CSF flow" study is not essential. Surgeons use it to obtain a baseline and gauge the amount obstruction of CSF flow by the tonsils. If a CMI/syringomyelia patient does not improve their symptoms after surgery, and the CSF flow is not improved it may change the management of that patient. Flow studies are also helpful for an uncommon entity called Chiari 0 malformation. These are patients with a syringomyelia but no cerebellum below the foramen magnum. The flow studies may demonstrate and obstruction of flow across the foramen magnum from something other than the tonsils, which causes the syringomyelia. Those patients can be improved with surgery.

Treatment

Treatment of CMI is primarily surgical as there is no effective medical treatment for this malformation [4]. However, the first and most important question is to determine whether or not surgery is required. In asymptomatic patients who may have borderline descent of their cerebellum (less than 5 mm), surgery may not be indicated for three reasons. The first reason is the patient's natural history may be one in which they stay asymptomatic throughout their life. Second, the MRI is a safe and cost effective tool to follow asymptomatic patients. And three, even in the most experienced and skilled neurological surgeons hands, the CMI operation is not without risks, albeit the risks may be low. So, who should get the surgery? The surgery is indicated for patients who have, (1) lifestyle limiting symptoms such as tussive headaches with a CMI on

MRI, (2) patients with neurological deficits attributed to their CMI and/or syringomyelia and (3) the CMI patient who has an expanding syringomyelia, as that is often correlated with neurological deterioration, (4) patients who have congenital skull base and cervical issue with resultant spinal instability or (5) hydrocephalus which is the cause of the downward herniation of the tonsils. The rare patients with spinal instability often require spinal fusion procedures and the rare patients with hydrocephalus often require a shunt procedure.

There are a wide variety of techniques that neurological surgeons perform CMI decompression surgery in the overwhelming majority of patients who do not have (4) or (5). The surgery rarely has to be performed in an emergency or urgent fashion unless the patient is experiencing progressive neurological deficits such as an expanding syringomyelia. However, the principles of the surgery are quite similar despite nuances in techniques between surgeons.

The two main goals of surgery for CMI is to (1) give the cerebellum, brainstem and spinal cord more room and (2) return the CSF flow in the back of the brain to as normal as possible. The surgery consists of removing a piece of bone in the back of the skull and upper spinal canal to increase the space, which in turn permits more normal CSF flow above and below the foramen magnum. To increase the space the neurological surgeon will usually remove a portion of the C1 vertebra (the lamina), the uppermost bone in the spine and remove a small piece of bone at the base of the skull in the back of the head to include the rim of the foramen magnum. Removing the rim of the foramen magnum and C-1 lamina permits the cerebellum to sit more comfortably in that space and facilitates more normal CSF flow around the cerebellum. This does not cause spinal instability. Often the dura, which is the covering of the cerebellum and brain, is opened and a patch of tissue is sewn in to expand the space which helps restore more normal CSF flow. The patch of tissue sewn into the dura to expand the space can be taken from the patient's native tissue under the scalp or sterile synthetic material. Sometimes the surgeon has to remove scar or shrink the tonsils with electro cautery to facilitate more CSF flow before the patch is sewn in place. The surgical manipulation of the tonsils does not cause any brain dysfunction; it alleviates and pre-empts adverse symptoms related to the cerebellar malformation. Additionally, this surgery when successful, also leads to the shrinkage of syringomyelia when present. The decrease in the diameter of a syringomyelia cystic dilation is essential to improve the function of the spinal cord. The CMI surgery is considered successful with most of the tussive headache symptoms improve and the neurological symptoms from the CMI and syringomyelia (when present) lessen because the syrinx cyst starts to collapse. When the correct surgical indications are applied by an experienced surgeon to a patient with a CMI or a CMI with syringomyelia, the overwhelming majority of the patients improve to some degree.

Immediately post-operatively, the patient requires pain medications because to access the skull in the back of the head the surgeons must dissect through the very well developed muscles that hold up the skull. Patients are out of bed walking the day after surgery and home several days after that. Patients should not return to vigorous athletic activity for 3 months after the surgery in order to permit the wound to heal and the patient to rebuild their endurance. Patients who undergo placement of a dura patch can suffer a leak of CSF for a host of reasons, which include over vigorous activity, which raise the pressure in the brain, but that complication is fortunately not common. There will be considerable discomfort for the patient initially but that slowly disappears as the patient heals. In the first month following the operation light activity is encouraged, however the patient is to avoid heavy lifting or similar strenuous activity so that they do not risk a CSF leak. The patient may also be prescribed a laxative to avoid strenuous bowel movements following surgery, as narcotic medications have been known to cause constipation. Any sign of infection around the surgical wound such as redness, tenderness, or purulence (presence of pus), is cause for immediate concern and should be reported to the treating physician as soon as possible.

In summary the CMI with or without syringomyelia is a surgically treatable disease. The outcome is usually quite good in experienced surgeons hands, and in patients who truly require the surgery because of lifestyle limiting pain, syringomyelia and/or neurological dysfunction.

References

1. Armonda RA, Citrin CM, Foley KT, Ellenbogen RG. Quantitative cine-mode MRI of chiari I malformations: an analysis of CSF dynamics. Neurosurgery. 1994;35(2):214–24. PMID: 7969828.
2. Toldo I, Tangari M, Mardari R, Perissinotto E, Sartori S, Gatta M, Calderone M, Battistella PA. Headache in children with chiari I malformation. Headache. 2014;54:899–908. doi:10.1111/head.12341.
3. Milhorat TH, Chou MW, Trinidad EM, Kula RW, Mandell M, Wolpert C, Speer MC. Chiari I malformation redefined: clinical and radiographic findings for 364 symptomatic patients. Neurosurgery. 1999;44:1005–17.
4. Ulrich B, editor. Chiari malformation and syringomyelia. American Syringomyelia and Chiari Alliance Project. Web. 26 June 2014. - http://asap.org/index.php/disorders/patient-handbook/.

Chapter 8
Brain Aneurysms

Yi Jonathan Zhang, Virendra Desai, Orlando Diaz, Richard P. Klucznik, and Gavin Britz

Introduction

Aneurysms are focal, weakened dilations of blood vessel walls. Most common aneurysms occur in the brain or along the aorta, where aneurysms affecting those vessels supplying the brain are called cerebral aneurysms. These dangerous dilations can cause life threatening bleeding from aneurysmal rupture and occasionally lead to symptoms by compressing adjacent neural structures. Many times, the very first bleeding from a brain aneurysm may lead to death. After rupturing once, aneurysms have a very high chance of rerupturing and rebleeding. Therefore, urgent treatment is of paramount importance in saving a salvageable patient's life. When a brain aneurysm is detected before any bleeding, careful evaluation should be made to determine whether and how to treat the potentially devastating abnormality.

Y.J. Zhang, MD
Department of Neurosurgery, Methodist Neurological Institute, Houston, TX, USA

V. Desai, MD • O. Diaz, MD • R.P. Klucznik, MD • G. Britz, MD (✉)
Department of Neurosurgery, Houston Methodist Hospital, Houston, TX, USA
e-mail: gbritz@houstonmethodist.org

A. Agrawal, G. Britz (eds.), *Emergency Approaches to Neurosurgical Conditions*, DOI 10.1007/978-3-319-10693-9_8,
© Springer International Publishing Switzerland 2015

Epidemiology

Before any symptom onset, most patients are not aware that they have an aneurysm. The prevalence of unruptured cerebral aneurysms in the general adult population ranges from 1.8 to 3.2 % [1, 2]. Of these, the overall risk of rupture is 1 % per year, although this risk depends significantly on age, type of aneurysm (symptomatic versus asymptomatic), size and location of the aneurysm [3]. In the U.S., there are approximately 30,000 cases of aneurysmal bleeding annually [4].

Pathophysiology

Much research has been devoted to the causes of brain aneurysm genesis. Currently, aneurysms are believed to form by a combination of weakness in the blood vessel wall and excessive pressure from within pushing outward on the wall. The primary cause of vessel wall weakness is atherosclerosis, although other causes such as infection and genetics exist [5]. Excessive pressure from within the vessel wall occurs in hypertensive patients, and generally, branching points of blood vessels are exposed to the highest blood pressures, predisposing these areas to aneurysm formation.

Unusual "mycotic aneurysms" can form when the blood vessel wall is weakened from ongoing infection or inflammation. This typically occurs in the setting of bacterial infection of the heart valves. Small packets of bacteria, called "septic emboli", arise from the heart and lodge in the blood vessel wall, leading to formation of an aneurysm [6].

Risk Factors

Risk factors for cerebral aneurysms can be divided into those that are modifiable and non-modifiable. Modifiable risk factors include cigarette smoking, certain medications, heavy alcohol consumption, and hypertension. Nonmodifiable risk factors include age, female sex, family history and hereditary disorders such as polycystic kidney disease and Ehlers Danlos syndrome [2, 7]. For instance, while a patient has the power to reduce or cease smoking cigarettes, they cannot change their age or gender.

Symptoms of Compression

Some aneurysms cause symptoms by compressing adjacent structures. Most commonly, this occurs with compression of the third cranial nerve, which controls the pupil as well as some eye muscles. This can cause double vision, a droopy eyelid and restricted eye movement [6]. Sometimes, aneurysms can grow very large, causing local swelling of the brain.

Symptoms of Rupture and Bleeding

When an aneurysm ruptures, it bleeds into a certain location within the skull known as the subarachnoid space, causing a "subarachnoid hemorrhage". When this occurs, patients present with headache, nausea, vomiting, neck stiffness, loss of consciousness or coma [6]. At times, before a catastrophic hemorrhage occurs, aneurysms leak a tiny amount, called a "sentinel bleed", causing headache, dizziness and vision changes [6]. After aneurysmal rupture, the patient's neurologic status can decline secondary to two processes: hydrocephalus or vasospasm. Hydrocephalus, literally "water in the head", occurs when the blood obstructs the flow and absorption of cerebrospinal fluid, which surrounds the brain and serves mainly as structural support. Vasospasm is a state of contraction and narrowing of blood vessels. The blood breakdown products from aneurysmal rupture can irritate the blood vessel wall, causing it to constrict. This obstructs blood flow downstream and can lead to stroke [6].

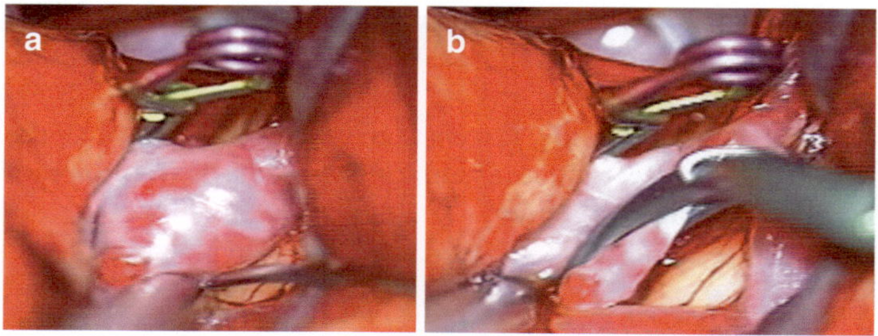

FIGURE 8.1 (**a**) This image depicts a gross, intra-operative view of a cerebral aneurysm in the center of the picture. At the sides of the aneurysms (*red color*) is the brain tissue. (**b**) This image shows a metallic clip about to be placed around the aneurysm (surgical clipping), sealing it off from the circulation

Diagnosis

Aneurysms are diagnosed by imaging studies. The best imaging modality is cerebral angiogram, which involves placement of a catheter into an artery in the groin and guiding it up to blood vessels in the neck that supply the brain. Then contrast is injected, allowing visualization of the blood vessels and any associated abnormalities, such as aneurysms (Figs. 8.2, 8.3, 8.6, 8.7, 8.8, 8.9, 8.10 and 8.11). Other imaging techniques include computed tomography angiography (CTA) (Figs. 8.4 and 8.5) and magnetic resonance angiography (MRA), which are essentially CT and MRI scans focused on blood vessel anatomy. The advantage of CTA and MRA over catheter-guided angiography is that they are not invasive; however, they are less sensitive in detecting smaller aneurysms [8] and only provide static information.

Conventional Treatment

To prevent an aneurysm from rupturing, either primarily or secondarily after initial bleeding, surgeons may occlude the aneurysm either via open brain surgery or catheter-guided

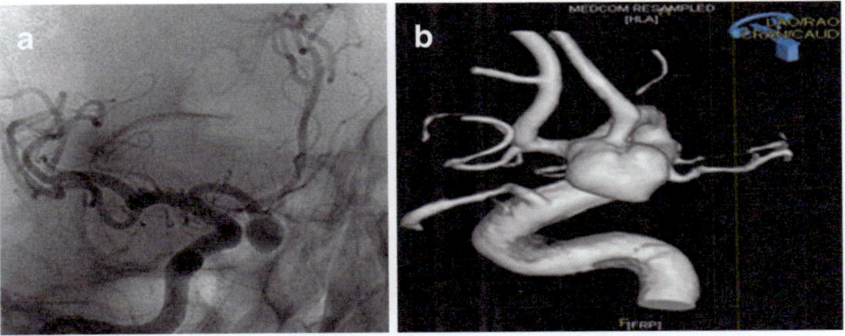

FIGURE 8.2 (**a**) 65 year-old with a large anterior communicating artery aneurysm with a cerebral angiogram of cerebral arteries when viewed from the front, showing a large aneurysm in the anterior communicating portion of the anterior cerebral arteries. (**b**) 3D reconstruction software takes pictures from a cerebral angiogram and creates an image similar to this, to better characterize the size and location of the aneurysm

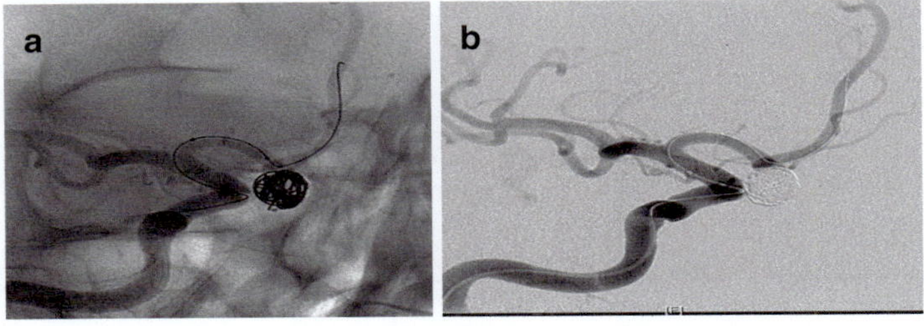

FIGURE 8.3 (**a**) The aneurysm depicted in Fig. 8.2 has now been coil embolized – note the dark coils placed inside the aneurysm. (**b**) Another view of the aneurysm in Fig. 8.2 after coil embolization

therapy. The former is referred to as "clipping" of an aneurysm while the latter is termed "endovascular coiling" or "embolization" [9].

Clipping involves placing a metallic clip at the base of the aneurysm, sealing it off from normal circulation so that blood cannot enter it and leak out (Figs. 8.1 and 8.5). Endovascular coiling involves placing platinum coils inside

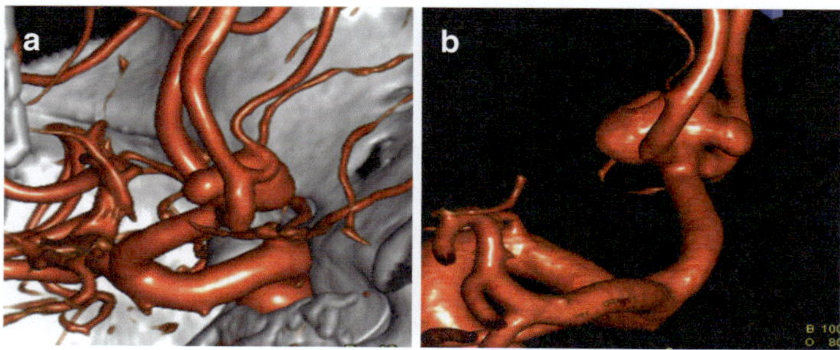

Figure 8.4 (**a**) 61 year-old female with subarachnoid hemorrhage secondary to ruptured anterior communicating aneurysm. 3D reconstruction of large anterior communicating artery aneurysm when viewed from the right side. (**b**) 3D reconstruction of large anterior communicating artery aneurysm when viewed from the left side

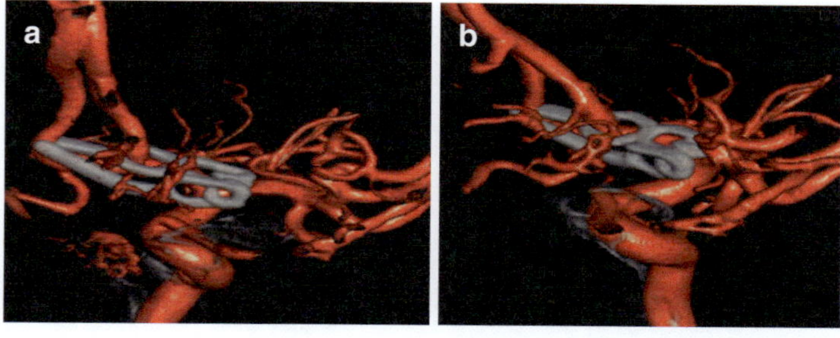

Figure 8.5 (**a**) The aneurysm in Fig. 8.4 has now been treated with a clip (front view). Note the jaws of the clip have an "open" portion that allows it to wrap around one of the anterior cerebral arteries without occluding it and still seal off the aneurysm (***keep image aspect ratio when enlarge***). (**b**) Same aneurysm after clip ligation when viewed from the side

the aneurysm pouch which promote the formation of blood clots, obliterating the aneurysm [9] (Fig. 8.3). Choosing the optimal therapy depends on many factors, including the patient's age and presenting symptoms, location, size and configuration of the aneurysm [9] and available expertise. Endovascular coiling was recently shown to have lower pro-

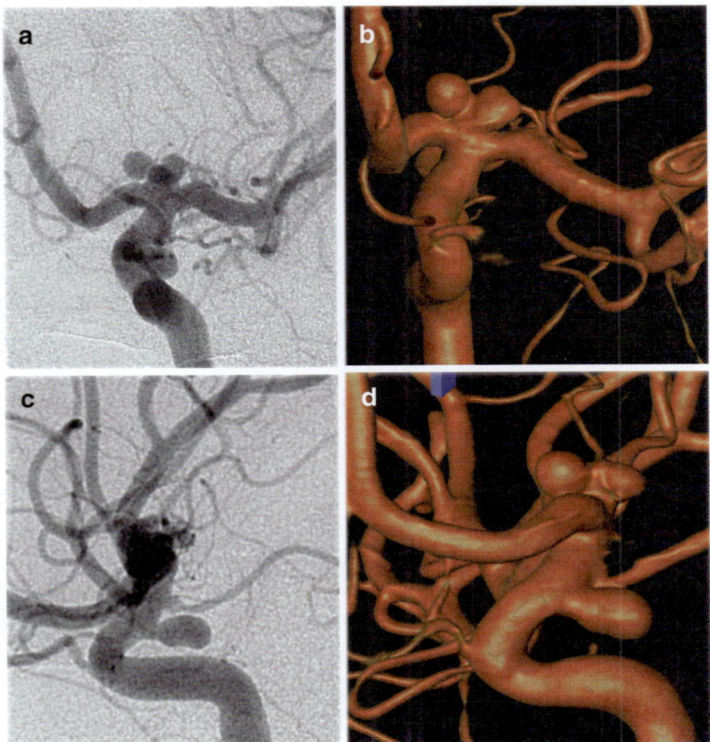

FIGURE 8.6 (a) 28 year-old male with subarachnoid hemorrhage found to have multiple left internal carotid artery aneurysms. Cerebral angiogram (front view) showing bilobed aneurysm at the very end of the internal carotid artery where it bifurcates into the anterior and middle cerebral arteries as well as a more proximal aneurysm projecting backwards off the internal carotid artery. (b) 3D reconstruction of the cerebral angiogram again showing the bilobed aneurysm at the end of the internal carotid artery. The aneurysm projecting backwards is not easily seen in this view. (c) Cerebral angiogram (side view) showing more clearly the aneurysm that projects backwards off the internal carotid artery. (d) 3D reconstruction of the cerebral angiogram (side view) showing both the bilobed aneurysm at the end of the internal carotid artery and the more proximal aneurysm that projects backwards off the internal carotid artery

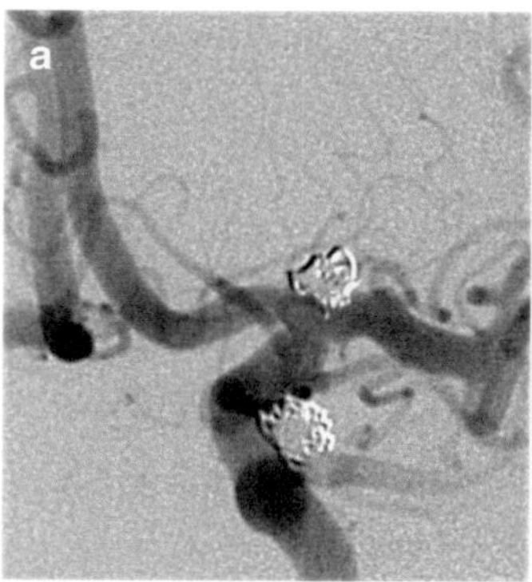
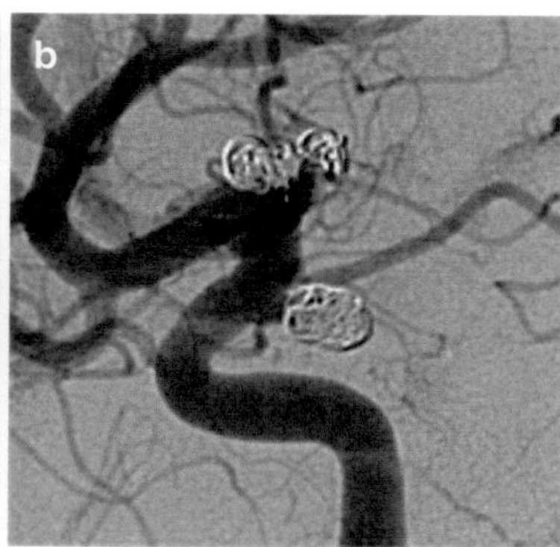

Figure 8.7 (**a**) Cerebral angiogram of the images in Fig. 8.6 after coil embolization of the aneurysms (front view). (**b**) Cerebral angiogram of the images in Fig. 8.6 after coil embolization of the aneurysms (side view)

cedural morbidity and mortality relative to surgical clipping. However, coiling also has a significantly higher rate of aneurysm recurrence. These facts play into the decision-making process, and each patient benefits from individualized assessment [8, 10].

Advanced Treatments: Stent Reconstruction, Flow Diversion, and Surgical Bypass

Some aneurysms are very complex due to their geometry and location, such that neither direct clipping nor endovascular coiling can be safely and/or effectively performed. Many new techniques and technologies have been developed in the past decade to address these challenges.

On the endovascular front, devices like balloons (Figs. 8.3 and 8.7) and stents (Figs. 8.10 and 8.11) can temporarily or permanently reconstruct the vessel wall at the inlet of an aneurysm, facilitating coiling of the defect. Most recently, a new class of stent, called flow diverters, can significantly change the blood flow pattern of the aneurysm, leading to

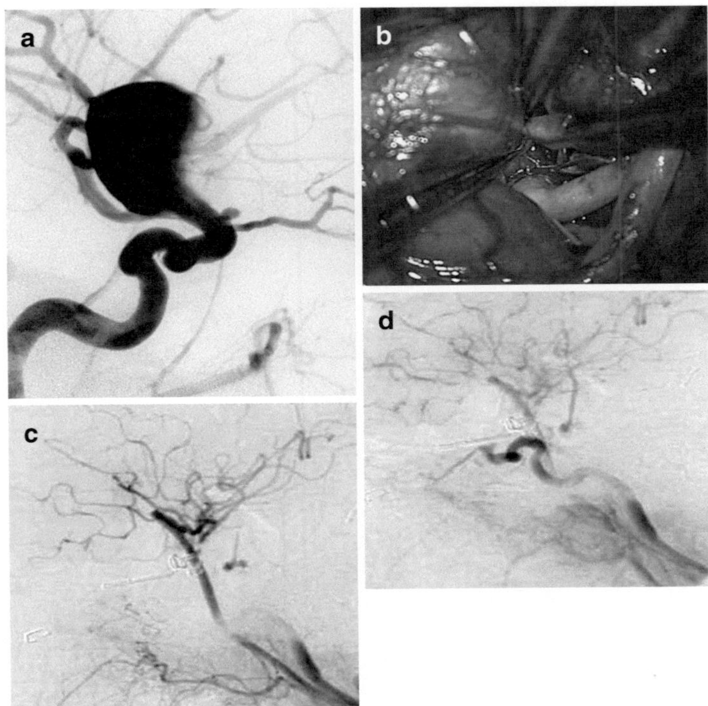

FIGURE 8.8 (**a**) 63 year-old woman suffered ruptured giant carotid aneurysm, angiogram in lateral view. This aneurysm cannot be treated with either coiling or direct clipping. (**b**) Intra-operative photo of bypass (pink tubular structure in right corner) to provide alternate blood flow into the brain from neck; followed with permanent aneurysm occlusion. (**c**) Intra-operative angiogram to show the bypass (dark lower center vessel) supplying the whole left brain. (**d**) Intra-operative angiogram to show complete occlusion of the aneurysm

promises of more durable endovascular occlusion. When using stents or flow diverters, patients have to take blood thinners, particularly clopidogrel (Plavix), to prevent clot formation on the devices. Hence, their use in the setting of acute bleeding may be limited.

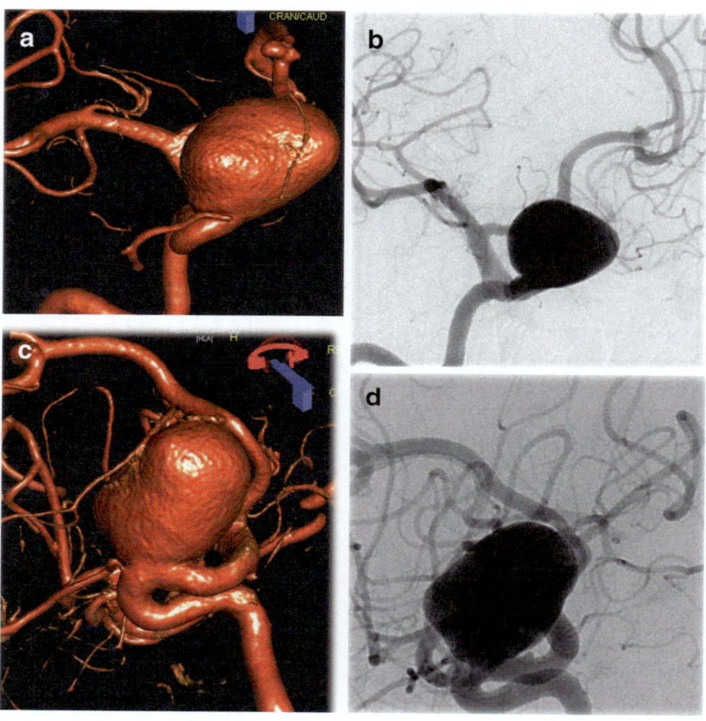

FIGURE 8.9 (**a**) 62 year-old suffered vision loss and was found to have a right ophthalmic artery aneurysm. 3D reconstruction of a giant ophthalmic artery aneurysm (front view). (**b**) Cerebral angiogram of a giant ophthalmic artery aneurysm (front view). (**c**) 3D reconstruction of a giant ophthalmic artery aneurysm (side view). (**d**) Cerebral angiogram of a giant ophthalmic artery aneurysm (side view)

On the surgical front, a technique to re-route blood flow to or within the brain can be used to manage very difficult, usually very large, aneurysms. This is called bypass surgery (Fig. 8.8a–d). It has been increasingly used as a tool to minimize the risks of stroke during aneurysm surgery. With this method, the newly-built vessel connection can allow prolonged or permanent occlusion of the artery on which the aneurysm resides, while the downstream brain tissue

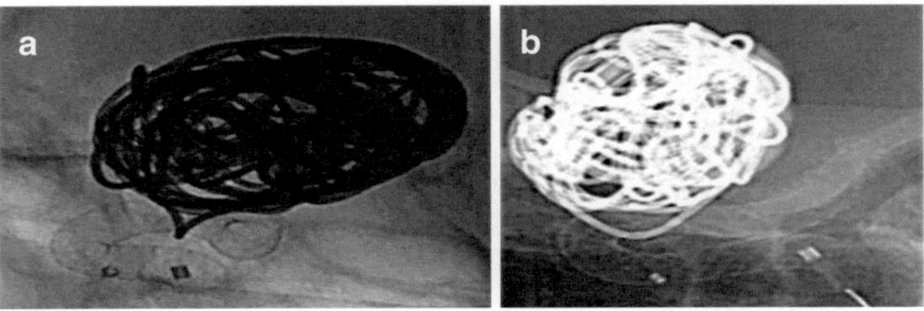

FIGURE 8.10 (**a**) Cerebral angiogram of the images in Fig. 8.9 after coil embolization of the aneurysm with the help of a pipeline stent, which can be noted as the smaller c-shaped structure contained within the internal carotid artery below the aneurysm (close-up view). (**b**) Cerebral angiogram of the images in Fig. 8.9 after coil embolization of the aneurysm with the help of a pipeline stent, which can be noted as the smaller c-shaped structure contained within the internal carotid artery below the aneurysm (close-up view)

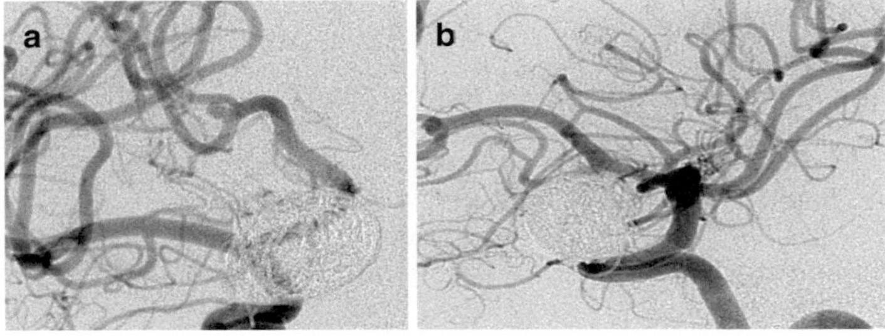

FIGURE 8.11 (**a**) Cerebral angiogram frontal view of Pipeline-treated giant aneurysm, 6-month after the treatment, which showed complete healing of the vessel and "disappearance of aneurysm". (**b**) Cerebral angiogram lateral view of the same complete treatment result of the giant aneurysm

continues receiving blood flow via the bypass. Bypass surgery can be performed by connecting either a large artery outside the skull to another artery within the skull or by connecting two arteries within the skull to each other. Bypass surgery is technically highly challenging and requires neurosurgeons with special training and experience [11]. Use of these technologies and techniques complicates aneurysm treatment, and they are generally only offered in large academic medical centers for the most difficult aneurysms.

Prognosis

Before 1995 [5], after subarachnoid hemorrhage from a ruptured aneurysm, 50 % of patients died with another 20 % dependent on others for activities of daily living (such as cooking, cleaning, dressing oneself, etc.). Over the last decade, the outcome has improved significantly, although brain aneurysm rupture continues to be a devastating condition. The most important factors in predicting outcome is the patient's age and condition prior to treatment.

References

1. Vernooij MW, Ikram MA, Tanghe HL, Vincent AJPE, Hofman A, Krestin GP, Niessen WJ, Breteler MMB, van der Lugt A. Incidental findings on brain MRI in the general population. N Engl J Med. 2007;357:1821–8.
2. Vlak MHM, Algra A, Brandenburg R, Rinkel GJE. Prevalence of unruptured intracranial aneurysms, with emphasis on sex, age, comorbidity, country, and time period: a systematic review and meta-analysis. Lancet Neurol. 2011;10:626–36.
3. Rinkel GJE, Djibuti M, Algra A, van Gijn J. Prevalence and risk of rupture of intracranial aneurysms: a systematic review. Stroke. 1998;29:251–6.
4. Singer RJ, Ogilvy CS, Rordorf G. Etiology, clinical manifestations, and diagnosis of aneurysmal subarachnoid hemorrhage. UpToDate.com. Wolters Kluwer; 2012.
5. Ruigrok YM, Rinkel GJE. Genetics of intracranial aneurysms. Stroke. 2008;39:1049–55.
6. Moore SP, Psarros TG. The definitive neurological surgery board review. Marceline: Walsworth Publishing; 2005. Print.
7. Krex D, Schackert HK, Schackert G. Genesis of cerebral aneurysms – an update. Acta Neurochir. 2001;143:429–49.

 8. Hacein-Bey L, Provenzale JM. Current imaging assessment and treatment of intracranial aneurysms. AJR Am J Roentgenol. 2011;196:32–44.
 9. Greenberg MS. Handbook of neurosurgery. 7th ed. Tampa: Thieme; 2010. Print.
10. Molyneux A, Kerr R, Stratton I, et al. International Subarachnoid Aneurysm Trial (ISAT) of neurosurgical clipping versus endovascular coiling in 2143 patients with ruptured intracranial aneurysms: a randomized trial. Lancet. 2003;360:1267–74.
11. Chen L, Lang L, Zhou L, Song D, Mao Y. Bypass or not? Adjustment of surgical strategies according to motor evoked potential changes in large middle cerebral artery aneurysm surgery. World Neurosurg. 2012;77(2):398e1-6.

Chapter 9
Brain Arteriovenous Malformations

Andrew B. Shaw, Daniel S. Ikeda, Evan S. Marlin, and Ciarán J. Powers

Abbreviations

AVM	Arteriovenous malformation
CPR	Cardiopulmonary resuscitation
CT	Computed tomography
CTa	Computed tomography angiography
DCA	Diagnostic cerebral angiography
MRa	Magnetic resonance angiography
MRI	Magnetic resonance imaging

Introduction

Arteries and *veins* are pipes, or blood vessels, by which blood is circulated throughout the body. Blood serves to carry nutrients to tissues and organs and takes waste products away from them. The heart serves as the pump that circulates blood

A.B. Shaw, MD • D.S. Ikeda, MD • E.S. Marlin, MD
C.J. Powers, MD, PhD (✉)
Department of Neurological Surgery,
The Ohio State University's Wexner Medical Center,
N-1018 Doan Hall 410 West 10th Avenue,
Columbus, OH 43210, USA
e-mail: Andrew.shaw@osumc.edu; Daniel.ikeda@osumc.edu;
evan.marlin@osumc.edu; ciaran.powers@osumc.edu

A. Agrawal, G. Britz (eds.), *Emergency Approaches to Neurosurgical Conditions*, DOI 10.1007/978-3-319-10693-9_9,
© Springer International Publishing Switzerland 2015

through this complex system of pipes. Arteries are charged with carrying blood away from the heart to the body. These vessels have thicker walls with multiple layers of muscle and collagen. This layered system allows the vessels to tolerate higher pressures. In contrast, veins have thinner walls and are under lower pressure. As arteries approach the level of tissues their diameters progressively decrease in size until they become *capillaries*. Capillaries are the smallest blood vessels and connect arteries to veins. Their thin walls allow water, oxygen, nutrients, and waste to cross easily to and from the surrounding tissues.

An *arteriovenous malformation* (AVM) is an abnormal tangle of blood vessels where arteries connect directly to veins without this intervening bed of capillaries (Fig. 9.1). This results in a direct connection from a high-pressure system to a low-pressure system. AVMs can be found throughout the body, including the brain. Brain AVMs typically have a *nidus*, or compact tangle of abnormal vessels. There is no normal brain tissue within the nidus. AVMs are spontaneous lesions that tend to enlarge with age. A little more than 1 in 1,000 people harbors these lesions [1]. They occur slightly more frequently in males than females and are usually diagnosed in an individual's 30s. This chapter will focus on the symptoms, diagnosis, and treatment of brain AVMs.

Symptoms and Presenting Features

AVMs can present with a variety of symptoms depending on size, location, and if they have bled before. AVMs bleed, or *hemorrhage*, because of the abnormal vessels contained

FIGURE 9.1 In these side (**a**) and front (**b**) views of an artist's impression of a brain AVM, note the abnormal tangle of vessels, *nidus*, with feeding arterial vessels and draining veins (Courtesy, The Aneurysm and AVM Foundation. © 2013 The Aneurysm and AVM Foundation. All Rights Reserved)

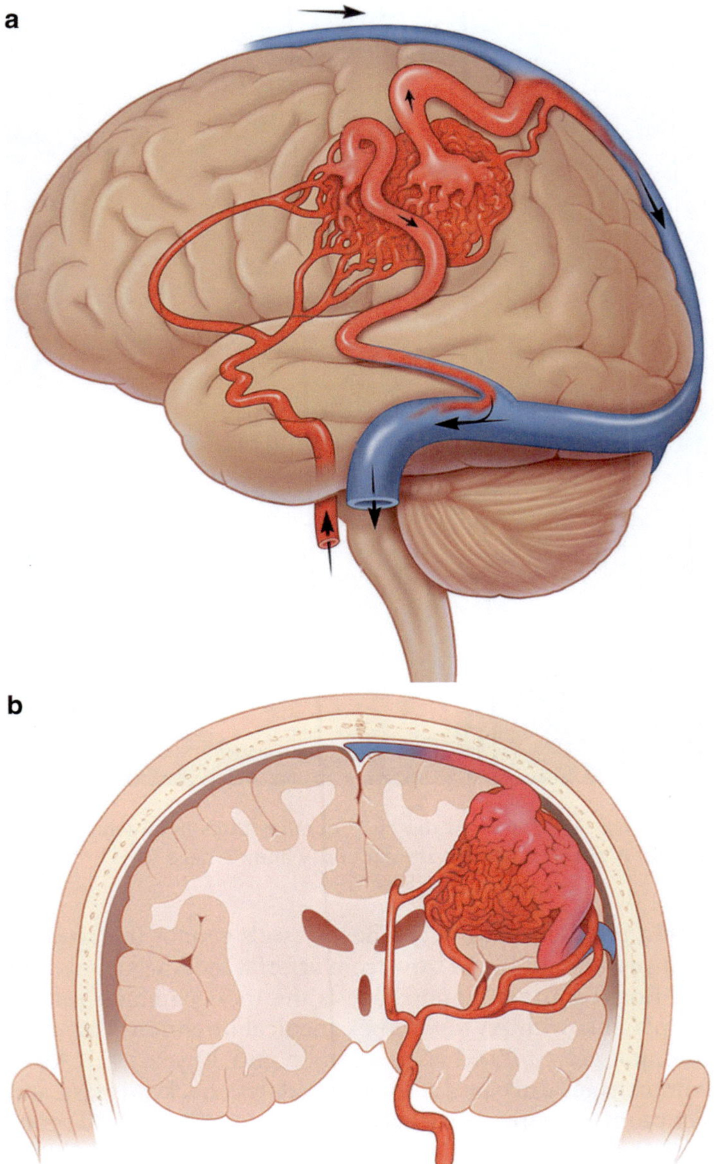

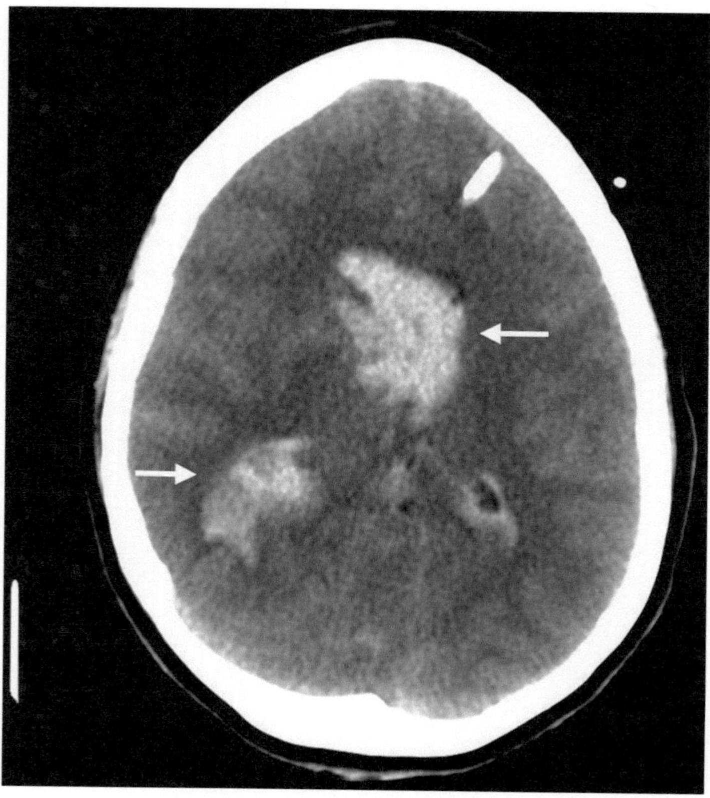

FIGURE 9.2 A CT scan of the head demonstrates hemorrhage from a brain AVM. The *white arrows* identify hemorrhage

within the nidus (Fig. 9.2). These vessels cannot tolerate the high-pressure of blood flow from arterial feeding vessels and can rupture. Brain hemorrhage is the most common reason for patients with AVMs to seek medical attention. The most common age to bleed is between 15 and 20 years [2]. AVM hemorrhages can cause seizures, headache, neck stiffness, and symptoms of a stroke, such as weakness, numbness, and problems speaking, depending on the location within the brain (Fig. 9.3). In the worst scenarios, hemorrhages can cause

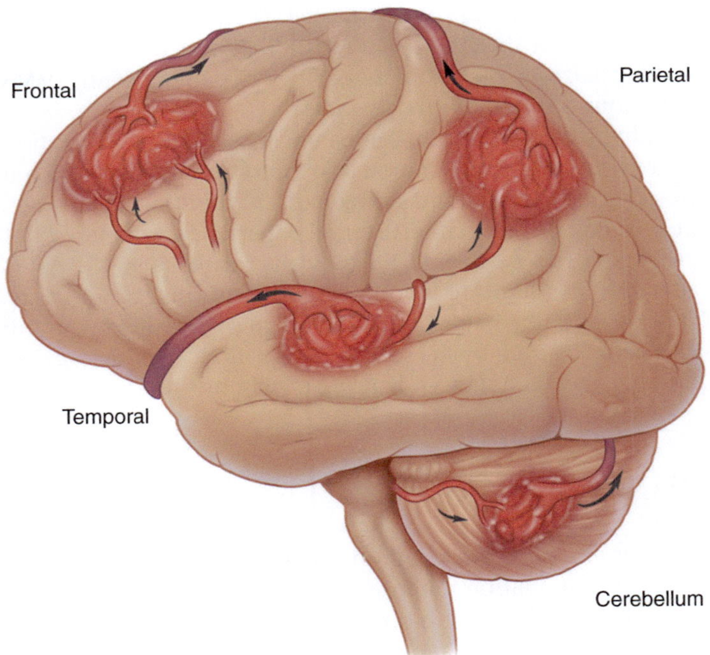

FIGURE 9.3 An illustration demonstrating the multiple locations brain AVMs can be found. AVM location is a critical factor in determining the possible risks of hemorrhage and risks from surgical removal (Courtesy, The Aneurysm and AVM Foundation. © 2013 The Aneurysm and AVM Foundation. All Rights Reserved)

coma or death. The exact risk of bleeding of brain AVMs is unknown, but believed to be between 2 and 4 % per year [3, 4]. The risk of bleeding may vary, depending on size and other features of the AVM [4, 5].

Seizure without hemorrhage is the second most common symptom leading to medical evaluation. A seizure results from abnormal electrical activity in the brain. A seizure can take a variety of forms including involuntary movements, altered level of consciousness, or muscle stiffness. Following a seizure the patient may be confused or sleepy. This is typically transient and will improve with time. The younger a patient is at diagnosis of the AVM, the more likely they will go on to develop seizures [3]. As many as 30 % of patients with AVMs may require treatment for seizures.

Individuals with these lesions may seek medical attention for a variety of other symptoms. Symptoms of increased brain pressure may develop including nausea, vomiting, headaches, and coma. Other patients may experience symptoms of stroke, or brain *ischemia*. This typically results from the AVM "stealing" or shunting blood away from normal brain tissue. This is often reversible. A more benign presenting symptom is a *bruit* caused by increased blood flow. In these cases, patients may complain of hearing a "whooshing" sound.

Diagnosis

Initially, emphasis is placed on previous medical history and physical examination in those seeking medical attention. This will guide the clinician to order the appropriate studies. In an emergency setting a *computed tomography* (CT) scan of the brain is obtained to look for evidence of bleeding. This technology utilizes "x-rays" to take snapshots of the body in cross sections. CT scans can be used to provide information about the vasculature by means of an intravenous dye called CT angiography (CTa) (Fig. 9.4). CT scans do have limitations in revealing details of the brain and requires exposure to radiation. In the setting of an AVM, it will allow doctors to identify bleeding, its source, and location, and it can be performed in conjunction with a CTa. Depending on the results, further diagnostic imaging studies may be obtained. This includes a *magnetic resonance imaging* (MRI) of the brain (Fig. 9.5). This imaging modality has the benefit of avoiding radiation and providing greater detail of the brain. This technology uses magnetic fields to differentiate different aspects of tissues. MRI has acquired new applications since its inception, and magnetic resonance angiography (MRa) can be performed. Similar to CTa, MRa provides information about

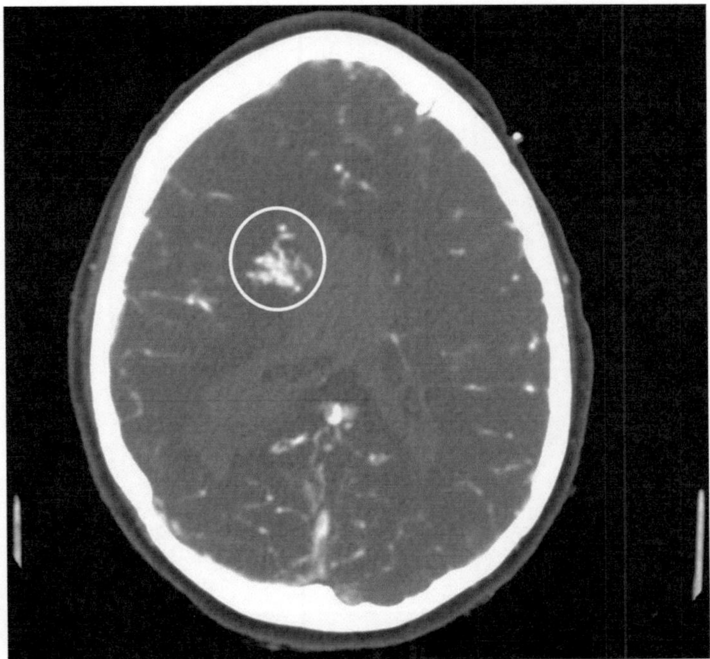

FIGURE 9.4 A CTa of the head demonstrates an AVM nidus (within the *white circle*) that is found as it takes up the contrast dye given intravenously and appears white on CTa

the blood vessels of the brain (Fig. 9.6). Information obtained from these studies will guide your physician in determining further evaluation or treatment.

Both CT and MRI technology are useful imaging studies to identify AVMs, however, the "gold standard" diagnostic study is a catheter-based *diagnostic cerebral arteriogram* (DCA). Typically, DCA is performed by making a small puncture in the femoral artery found in the groin. Through this puncture, a long, thin tube, or *catheter*, is navigated through blood vessels to the base of the brain. The arteries, *carotid and vertebral*, that travel to the brain are then injected with dye seen on x-ray as it flows through the blood vessels

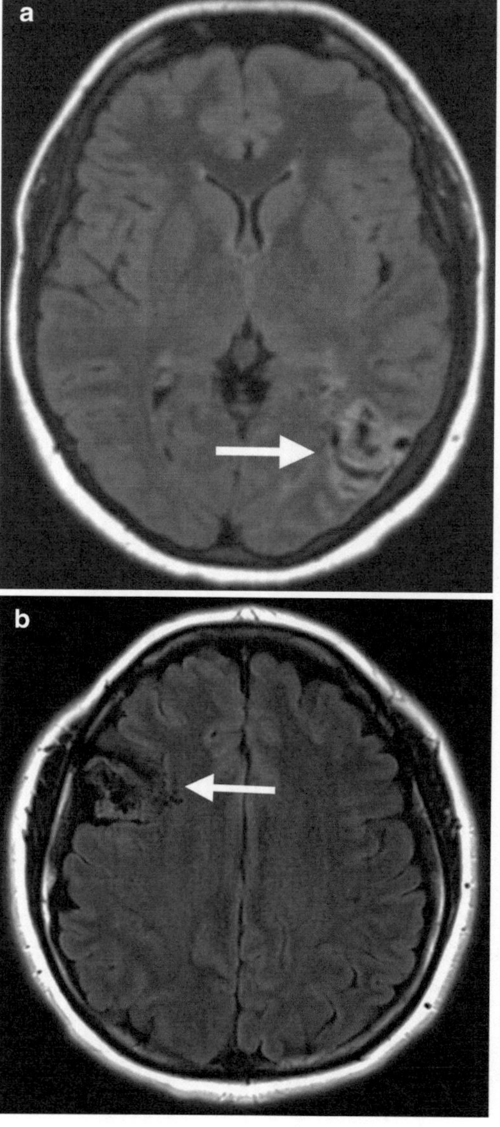

Figure 9.5 MR images (**a–c**) of three different patients with brain AVMs in different locations and sizes. The AVM nidus is demarcated by a *white arrow*

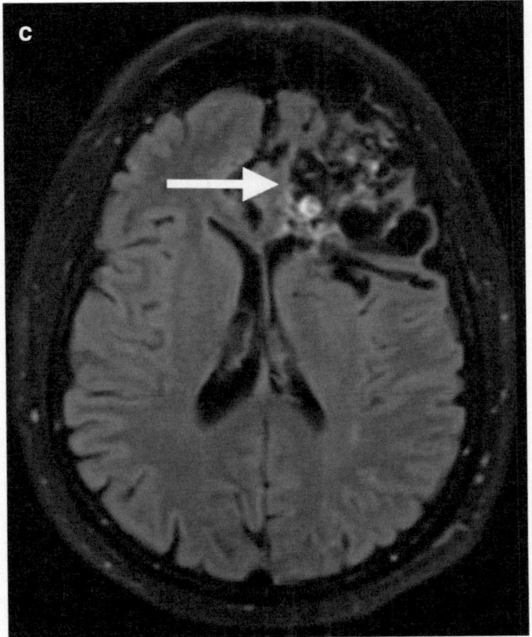

FIGURE 9.5 (continued)

and AVM (Fig. 9.7). The DCA can provide information about the AVM size, arterial inflow to the nidus, and venous outflow. This is an invasive study with risks of radiation, kidney injury from the dye, and blood vessel injury from the catheters, and is reserved for cases where the AVM needs to be better characterized after CT or MRI.

Treatment

A definitive measure to "cure" an individual of their AVM is surgical removal. Patients are put under general anesthesia and an incision in the scalp overlaying the brain AVM is made. After a "bone window", or craniotomy, is made to expose the underlying brain, the AVM is delicately

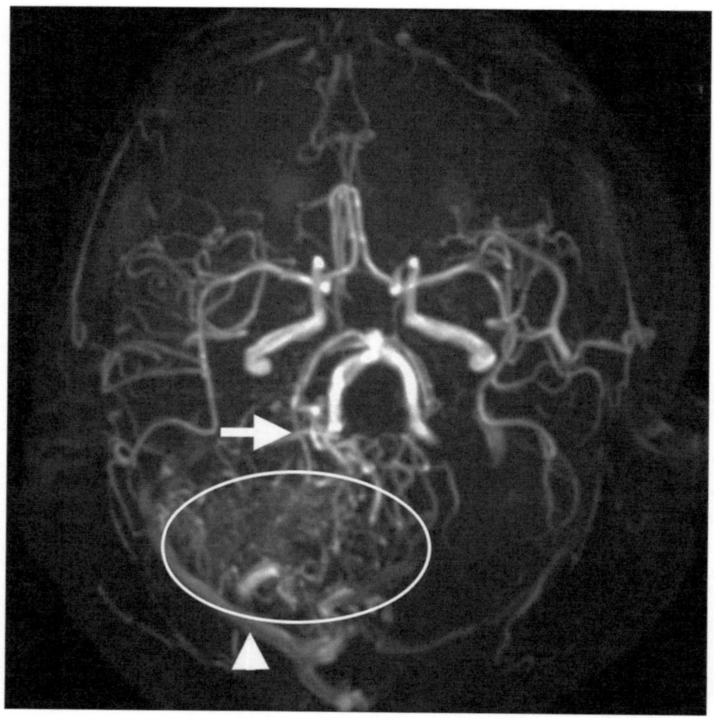

FIGURE 9.6 A MRa of a patient with a brain AVM demonstrates the feeding arteries (*white arrow*), the AVM nidus (*white ellipse*), and the draining vein (*white arrowhead*)

disconnected from the abnormal arterial and venous connections and removed. Care is taken not to injure surrounding brain structures (Fig. 9.8). Although surgery for AVMs offers the benefit of immediate cure, there are risks because of the invasive nature of surgery.

The treatment of AVMs has evolved over the last 20 years with new modalities that may decrease the risk of surgery or avoid it all together. Similar to the previously described DCA, a catheter-based treatment to decrease the blood flow through the AVM is often utilized as an adjunct to lessen blood loss during surgery and in rare cases is curative

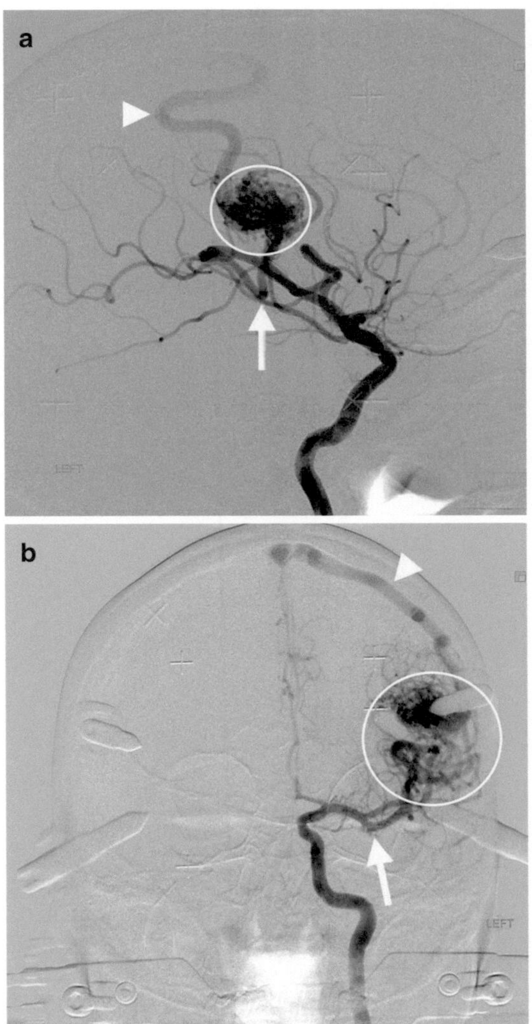

FIGURE 9.7 Images from side (**a**) and front (**b**) projections of a DCA demonstrate the feeding arteries (*white arrow*), the AVM nidus (*encircled*), and the draining vein (*white arrowhead*). This remains the "gold standard" diagnostic study

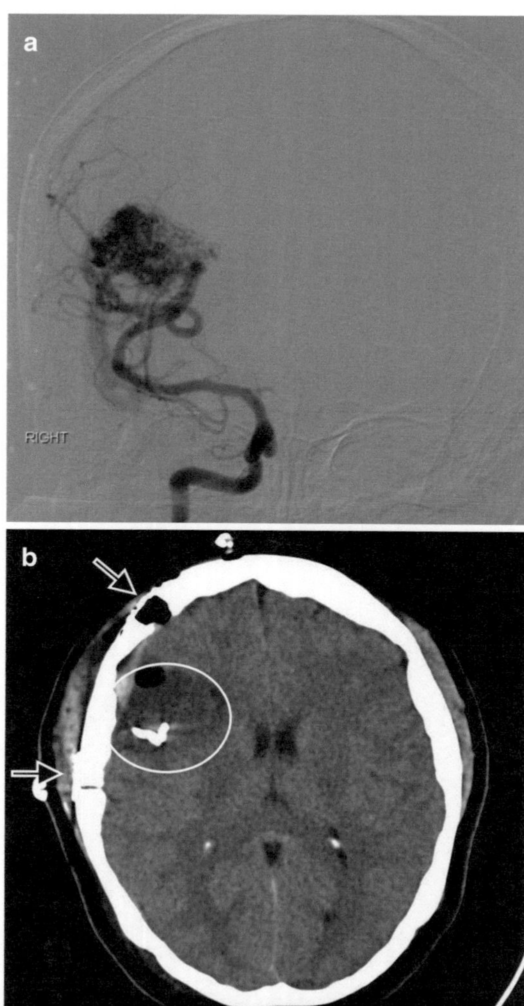

FIGURE 9.8 A DCA (**a**) performed before surgery demonstrates the AVM of a patient with significant uncontrolled seizures. A CT scan (**b**) performed immediately after surgery demonstrates the defect (*encircled*) from removing the AVM and evidence of a "bone window" or craniotomy repaired with small titanium plates (*black arrows with white trim*). (**c**) A DCA performed 6 months after surgery demonstrates complete resection and "cure" of the previously seen AVM

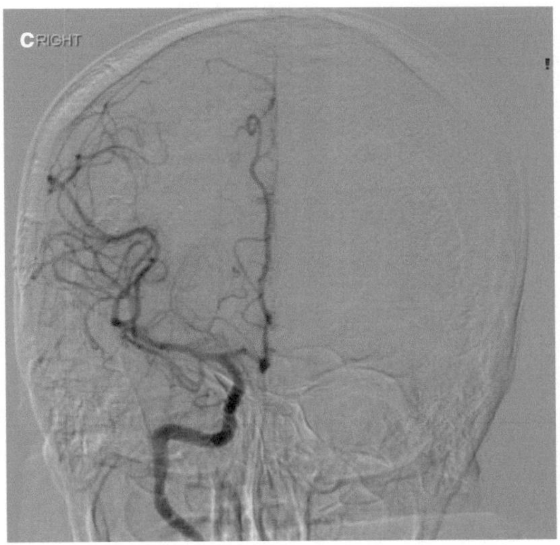

FIGURE 9.8 (continued)

(Fig. 9.9). Briefly, a catheter is brought into an abnormal feeding artery of the AVM nidus, and agents, similar to liquid cement, can be used to stop blood flow through *embolization* or plugging of the blood vessel [6]. Another modality that continues to evolve is radiation or *stereotactic radiosurgery* (Fig. 9.10), which uses concentrated x-rays to induce changes within the AVM, ultimately leading to closure of the abnormal vessels [7]. The benefit of this treatment includes its relative noninvasiveness. However, just as in the other modalities, there are risks associated with radiation therapy and may take 3 years to achieve a cure.

Seizures caused by the AVM are often treated with medications. Seizure frequency may change after treatment and the need for medications may change. A clinician may decide to treat an individual with any one or combination of these treatments. Some AVMs are not amenable to these treatments and continued observation may be the best option.

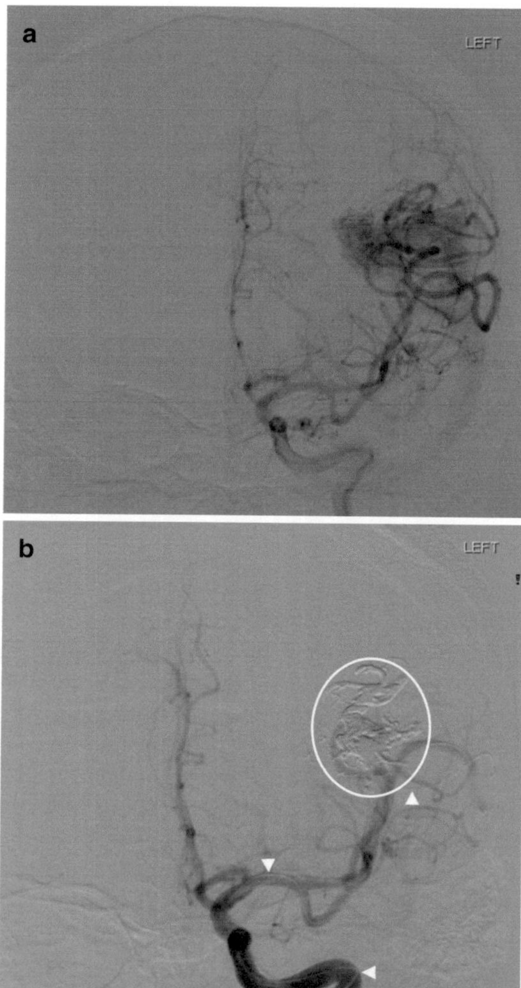

FIGURE 9.9 A DCA (**a**) demonstrates the classic appearance of an AVM nidus. A repeat DCA after *embolization* (**b**) demonstrates complete absence of filling of the nidus. Note the substance used to "plug" or embolize the AVM (*encircled*). This embolization agent, similar to liquid cement, is delivered to the AVM by a long, thin tube or catheter (*arrowheads*)

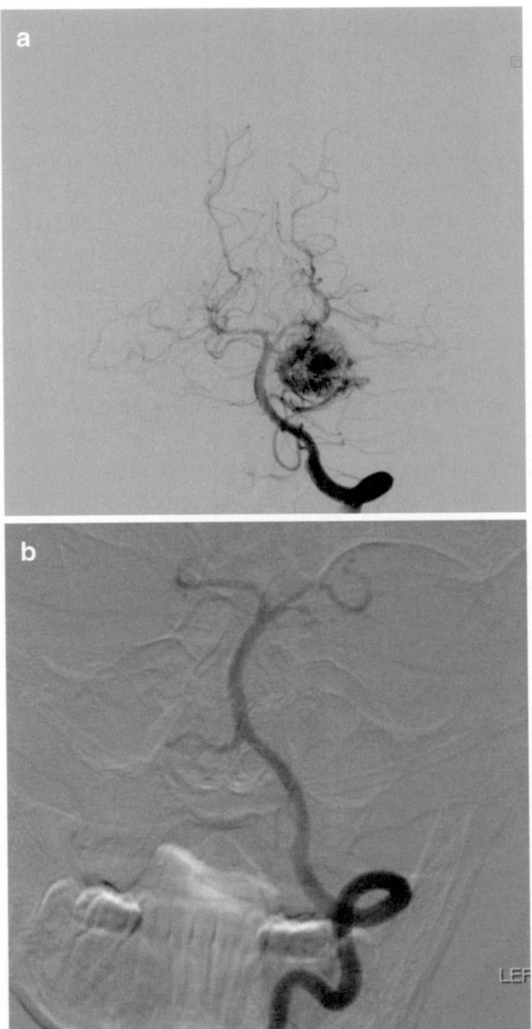

FIGURE 9.10 A DCA (**a**) demonstrates a fairly large AVM in the cerebellum, or hindbrain. This was treated with *stereotactic radiosurgery*. A repeat DCA (**b**) performed approximately 3 years later demonstrates complete absence of the AVM

Medical Emergencies Associated with Brain AVMS

Hemorrhage from an AVM is a medical emergency. If symptoms of bleeding present such as a worsening, atypical headache, altered mental status, or signs of stroke develop, emergency services should be contacted immediately. If the individual is unresponsive, someone trained in cardiopulmonary resuscitation (CPR) should assess the patient's level of consciousness, pulse rate, and ability to breathe. If no pulse or spontaneous breathing is found, CPR should be commenced until emergency services arrive.

Individuals known to harbor AVMs may have frequent seizures and families should be aware of this symptom. If someone is having a seizure you should first ensure that the patient is safe by removing objects that may be harmful. Do not attempt to put anything in their mouth. If a seizure lasts longer than 5 min, emergency services should be contacted. When someone "awakens" from a seizure, they are often confused. This is usually transient. Ensure the medication the individual takes for seizures is given to the emergency services or the clinician.

Conclusion

AVMs are rare lesions composed of abnormal connections between arteries and veins. Individuals with these lesions have variable symptoms and the prognosis varies depending on characteristics of the AVM. Diagnostic and therapeutic options continue to evolve, and treatment is individualized based on several factors. Patients with AVMs and their families should be aware of common symptoms and previous treatment in case of an emergency. This information is extremely useful in the emergency setting.

References

1. Ondra SL, Troupp H, George ED, Schwab K. The natural history of symptomatic arteriovenous malformations of the brain: a 24-year follow-up assessment. J Neurosurg. 1990;73:387–91.
2. Perret G, Nishioka H. Report on the cooperative study of intracranial aneurysms and subarachnoid hemorrhage. Section VI. Arteriovenous malformations. An analysis of 545 cases of craniocerebral arteriovenous malformations and fistulae reported to the cooperative study. J Neurosurg. 1966;25:467–90.
3. Crawford PM, West CR, Chadwick DW, Shaw MD. Arteriovenous malformations of the brain: natural history in unoperated patients. J Neurol Neurosurg Psychiatry. 1986;49:1–10.
4. Spetzler RF, Hargraves RW, McCormick PW, Zabramski JM, Flom RA, Zimmerman RS. Relationship of perfusion pressure and size to risk of hemorrhage from arteriovenous malformations. J Neurosurg. 1992;76:918–23.
5. Stapf C, Mast H, Sciacca RR, Choi JH, Khaw AV, Connolly ES, et al. Predictors of hemorrhage in patients with untreated brain arteriovenous malformation. Neurology. 2006;66:1350–5.
6. Amar AP, Teitelbaum GP, Larsen DW. A novel technique and new grading scale for the embolization of cerebral vascular malformations. Neurosurgery. 2006;59:S158–62; discussion S3–13.
7. Lunsford LD, Niranjan A, Kano H, Kondziolka D. The technical evolution of gamma knife radiosurgery for arteriovenous malformations. Prog Neurol Surg. 2013;27:22–34.

Chapter 10
Moyamoya Disease

Teresa E. Bell-Stephens and Gary K. Steinberg

Moyamoya Disease

Moyamoya causes progressive narrowing and closure in the intracranial ICAs and their branches (anterior and middle cerebral arteries). It usually affects both sides, but is sometimes unilateral [14, 24, 26]. The result is often temporary or permanent neurological symptoms including transient ischemic attacks (TIAs), strokes, headaches, seizures, abnormal uncontrolled movements and/or various other symptoms [23, 24, 31] (Table 10.1). Adults have a greater risk of stroke from bleeding than do children. Initially thought to be limited to those of Asian heritage, moyamoya is now recognized as affecting all ethnicities (Fig. 10.1). Once considered extremely rare, moyamoya diagnoses in the United States have increased with improved awareness. One study showed that 1 of every 200,000 hospital admissions in the United States was due to moyamoya, and this number has increased over time [27]. Symptoms can start at any age, but there are peaks in childhood around age 5 and in the fourth decade of life [26]. Some associated

T.E. Bell-Stephens, RN, BSN, CNRN • G.K. Steinberg, MD, PhD (✉)
Department of Neurosurgery, Stanford University School
of Medicine, 300 Pasteur Drive, Stanford, CA 94305-5327, USA
e-mail: tbell-stephens@stanfordhealthcare.org;
gsteinberg@stanford.edu

A. Agrawal, G. Britz (eds.), *Emergency Approaches to Neurosurgical Conditions*, DOI 10.1007/978-3-319-10693-9_10,
© Springer International Publishing Switzerland 2015

TABLE 10.1 Presenting symptoms of moyamoya patients at Stanford

Adults		Pediatric (<18 years)	
TIA	55 %	TIA	38 %
Stroke	59 %	Stroke	40 %
Hemorrhage	16 %	Hemorrhage	6 %
Seizure	14 %	Seizure	11 %
Headache	49 %	Headache	22 %

Ethnicity of moyamoya patients at Stanford

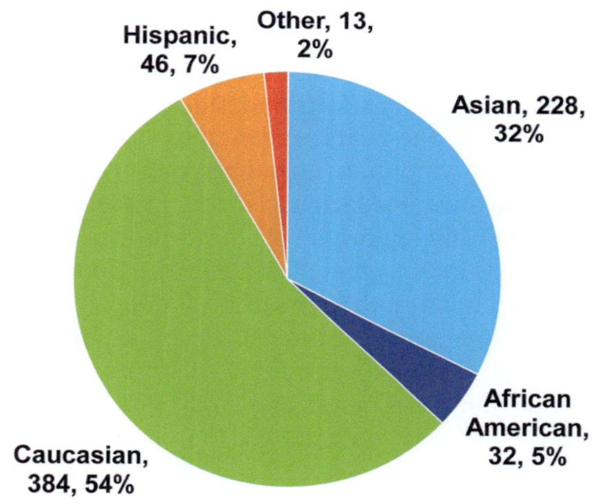

FIGURE 10.1 Ethnicity of the 703 moyamoya patients (1,132 revascularization procedures) treated at Stanford 1990–Feb 1, 2013

disorders also put patients at increased risk for developing moyamoya [8, 24, 26] (Table 10.2). Moyamoya occurs more commonly in females (Fig. 10.2) and they are more likely to have preoperative TIAs then men [15]. The reason for this is unknown, but it is not related to high cholesterol or other common stroke risk factors. Some cases are familial, and recently novel genes have been identified that predispose to developing moyamoya [2, 3, 11, 21].

TABLE 10.2 Disorders associated with moyamoya at Stanford

Disorder	Number of patients
Down syndrome	23
Neurofibromatosis	18
Graves' disease (hyperthyroid)	11
Sickle cell disease	6
Primordial dwarfism	6
Coarctation of the aorta	5
Post-radiation	5
Thalassemia	4
Morning Glory syndrome	2
Optic glioma	2
Alagille syndrome	1
G6PD deficiency	1
Glycogen storage disease	1
Hurler's disease	1
Lysosomal storage disease	1
MELAS syndrome	1
Noonan syndrome	1
Russell Silver syndrome	1
Systemic autoimmune disease	1
Wolff-Parkinson-White syndrome	1

Natural History

The natural history of moyamoya is not completely understood, although there is inevitable progression in the majority of patients. The rate of progression, however, is unpredictable. Two-thirds of patient have symptomatic progression over 5 years and the outcome is poor without treatment [6, 19, 20]. Those with unilateral presentation often

Gender of moyamoya patients at Stanford

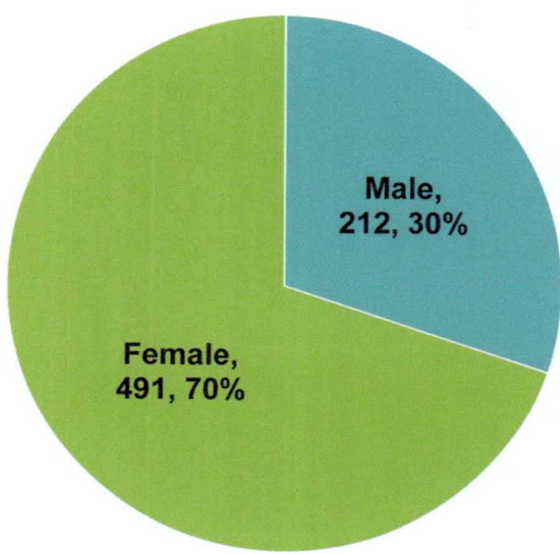

FIGURE 10.2 Gender of the 703 moyamoya patients (1,132 revascularization procedures) treated at Stanford 1990–Feb 1, 2013

develop moyamoya on the other side [14] and medical therapy alone is not effective in preventing progression. The 5-year stroke rate is 20–65 % with medical treatment only [5, 10, 28]. "Asymptomatic" moyamoya may not be entirely accurate [18], as 20 % of patients have silent infarcts (magnetic resonance imaging [MRI]-positive) and a 3.2 %/year stroke risk.

Diagnosis

Moyamoya diagnosis involves taking careful histories and evaluating several radiology studies. Patients are asked in-depth questions about the onset, frequency, location, duration and severity of any neurological symptoms in order to determine if they are related to moyamoya and which side of the brain might be affected. Moyamoya can initially be confused with other neurological disorders, such as multiple sclerosis [7],

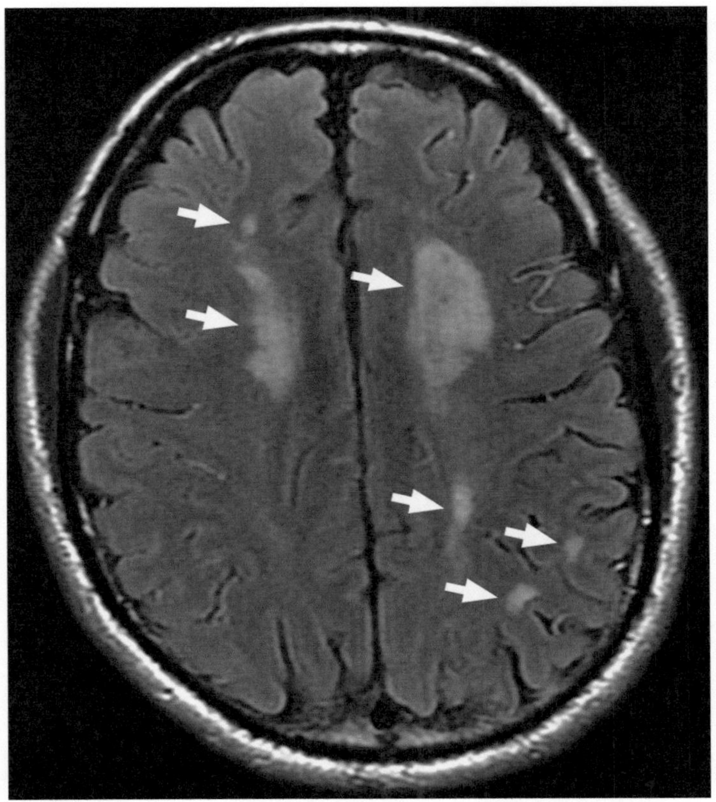

FIGURE 10.3 Preoperative MRI head scan showing strokes (*arrows*) on both sides of the brain secondary to moyamoya

until radiological studies confirm findings consistent with narrowing or closure of brain arteries.

MRI scans reveal brain structures and identify locations of infarcts or areas of bleeding (Fig. 10.3), MRI or computed tomography (CT) angiograms noninvasively screen blood vessels of the brain (Figs. 10.4 and 10.5) and cerebral angiograms show the structure of brain arteries (Fig. 10.6). Most common findings include narrowing or closure of the ICA or its branches. In addition, compensatory thin-walled arteries

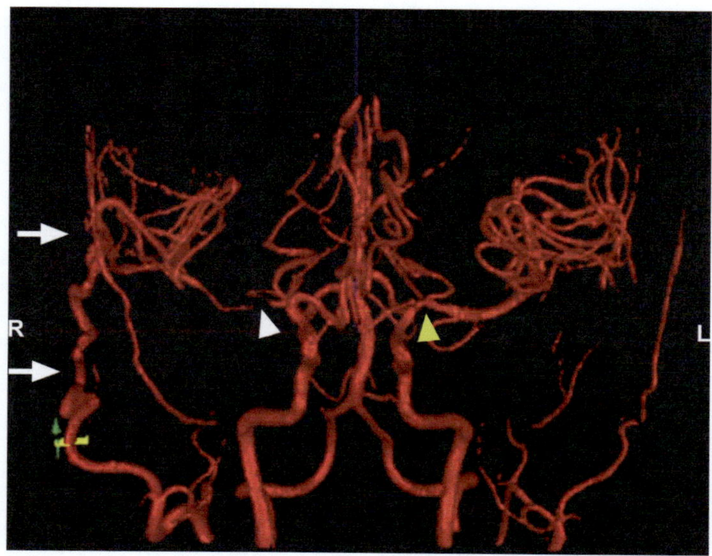

FIGURE 10.4 NOVA MRI shows flow through right STA-MCA bypass (*arrows*) filling the brain on the right side. Note the absence of the MCA on the right side (*white arrow head*) and mild narrowing of the MCA on left side (*yellow arrow*)

that develop over time may be present. These fragile "moyamoya" vessels, which led Japanese doctors to initially describe the "puff of smoke" appearance on angiograms [29], can bleed. If treatment is indicated, external carotid (scalp) arteries are examined to choose the best donor artery and the optimal technique for surgery.

Several different brain perfusion studies help determine how well blood vessels deliver oxygen to tissues of the brain. Patients may undergo one or more of these studies to evaluate brain perfusion, such as MRI, CT, PET and Xenon CT (Fig. 10.7) which, when combined with clinical history and physical evaluation, help guide treatment recommendations. Cognitive evaluation is also frequently done to assess for executive dysfunction (disorganization and impaired focus), which has been shown to be present at higher rates in adult moyamoya patients even without prior stroke [4, 12, 13].

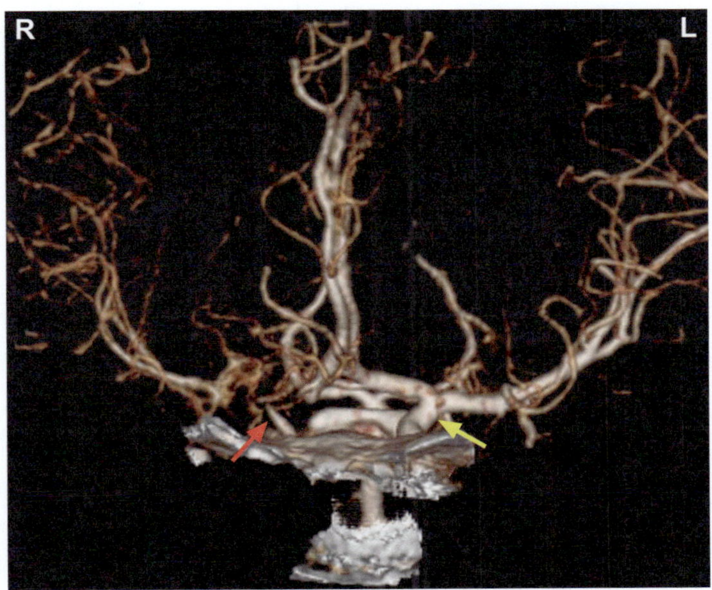

FIGURE 10.5 CT angiogram shows moyamoya on the right with closure of the ICA (*red arrow*) and a normal blood vessel on the left (*yellow arrow*)

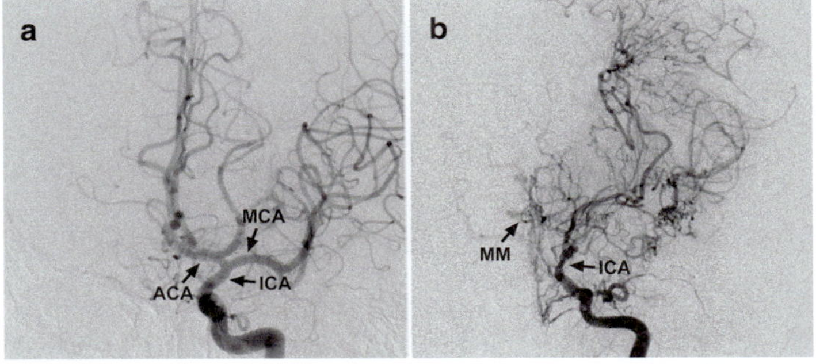

FIGURE 10.6 Cerebral angiogram. (**a**) Front view of a normal angiogram. (**b**) Front view of an angiogram showing moyamoya disease. Note the narrowing of the ICA and presence of moyamoya vessels. Also note the absence of the MCA and ACA. *ICA* internal carotid artery, *ACA* anterior carotid artery, *MCA* middle cerebral artery, *MM* moyamoya collateral arteries

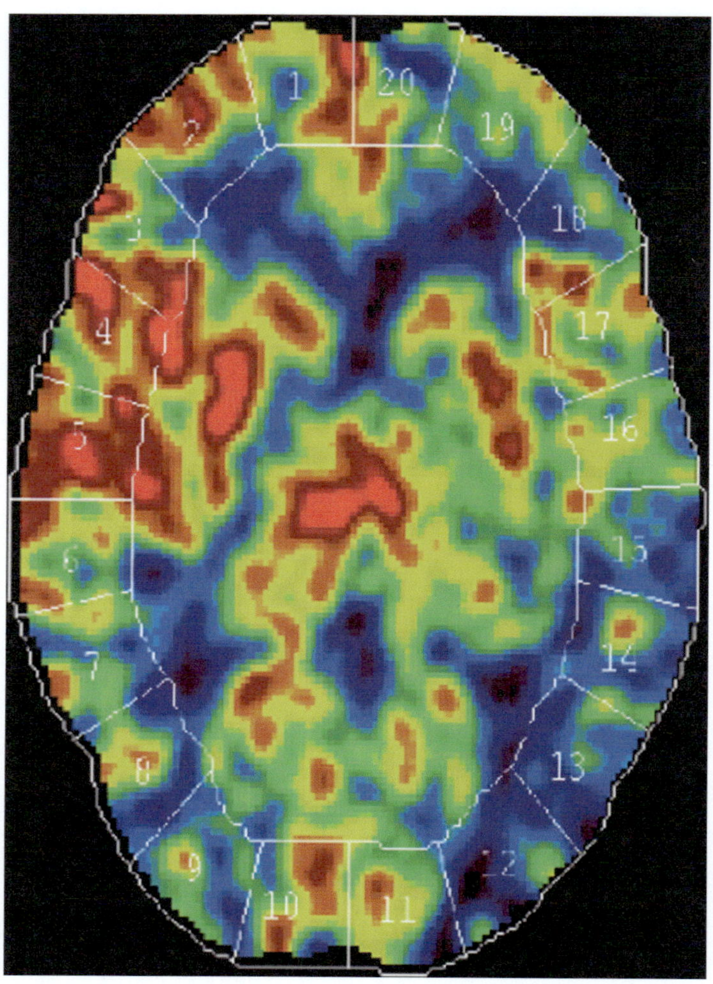

FIGURE 10.7 Xenon CT scan: This perfusion study shows reduced blood flow (*higher area of blue*) on the left side compared with normal perfusion on right side (*higher area of red*)

Treatment

Moyamoya is sometimes treated with antiplatelet or anticoagulation therapy in an attempt to improve blood flow to the brain. However, as previously mentioned, medical therapy alone is ineffective. The goal of treatment is to improve blood flow to the brain and prevent future stroke. Placement of stents, often effective against intracranial atherosclerosis, are ineffective against moyamoya long-term due to its lack of atherosclerotic etiology and progressive nature [16]. As most patients are young when moyamoya is diagnosed, surgery is usually recommended when symptomatic.

Surgical procedures include direct and indirect revascularization techniques. The direct bypass is known as the superficial temporal artery to middle cerebral artery (STA-MCA) bypass. This involves attaching a scalp artery (STA) directly into a brain artery (MCA) on the outer surface of the brain. Patients benefit from an immediate improvement in their blood flow when the bypass is completed as well as reduced risks of stroke. Indirect bypasses (encephalo-duro-synangiosis [EDAS], encephalo-duro-arterio-myo-synangiosis [EDAMS], pial synangiosis) involve placing a scalp artery or vascular muscle or tissue on the outer surface of the brain for gradual growth of blood supply inwards to areas in need. At least several months are required for ingrowth of new blood supply as well as stroke risk reduction using this method alone.

Determining which procedure to use at our institution is based on artery size at the time of surgery. Since 1990 Dr. Steinberg has performed 1,132 revascularization procedures in 703 moyamoya disease patients. Direct bypass is always the first option considered and, when possible, our preference is to perform a combined direct and indirect during the same surgery (Fig. 10.8). We reserve indirect revascularization procedures for young children (<5 years old) whose arteries are generally less than 7 mm in diameter or too fragile, making direct bypass less feasible [9].

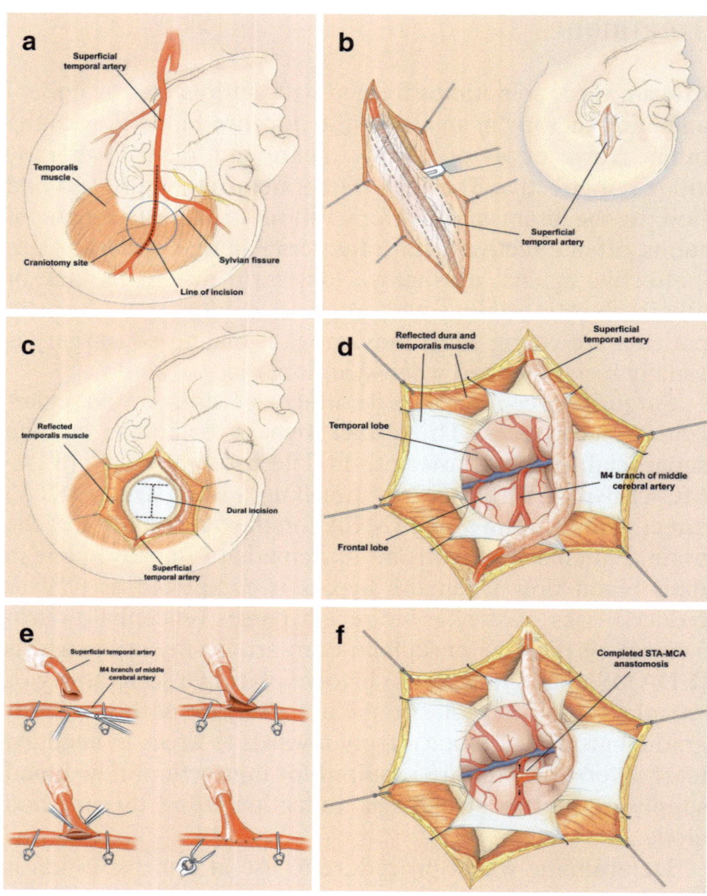

Figure 10.8 Diagram shows combined direct (*STA-MCA*) and indirect (EDAS) bypass: (**a, b**) STA (scalp) artery identified. (**c, d**) Small skull opening near bypass area and MCA (brain artery) identified. (**e**) STA sewn to MCA with soft tissue left on surrounding vessel for indirect bypass onlay of brain. (**f**) STA-MCA bypass in place with indirect bypass ready for onlay to surface of the brain (Reprinted from Guzman and Steinberg [9], Copyright (2010), with permission from Elsevier)

Patients with prior brain surgery may have no viable scalp arteries or temporalis muscle for bypass. In this case, indirect revascularization using omentum can be performed. Omental revascularization uses a rich vascular supply of tissue from the abdomen tunneled upwards and laid on the outer surface of the brain [22]. Microsurgical techniques, such as laparoscopic omental harvesting and tunneling, have substantially reduced the risks of this procedure.

What to Expect with Surgery

Each surgery lasts several hours, and patients are asleep for the entire procedure. After surgery, patients stay in the intensive care unit (ICU) overnight for close observation. Hospital stays vary, but are generally 2–3 days, during which time patients are expected to be as ambulatory as possible. Pain medication is given intravenously at first, and then given orally once patients are eating. After discharge, patients may tire more easily than usual for several weeks and often do not return to work or school for about 4 weeks. Specific instructions for activities are discussed with each individual patient. Skin staples or sutures remain for 7–10 days, and incision care is minimal and discussed at hospital discharge (Fig. 10.9). Dissolvable skin sutures are used in children. We recommend that patients avoid strenuous physical exercise for 4 weeks after surgery, but strongly encourage frequent walking.

Moyamoya and Lifestyle Implications

Moyamoya patients have very few lifestyle limitations. Lifelong antiplatelet medication, such as daily aspirin, is recommended to optimize flow through the bypass. Side effects from aspirin can include excessive bruising, bleeding and stomach irritation. Your doctor should be notified if this occurs. Artificial hormones, including birth control pills and hormone replacement therapy, should be avoided. These

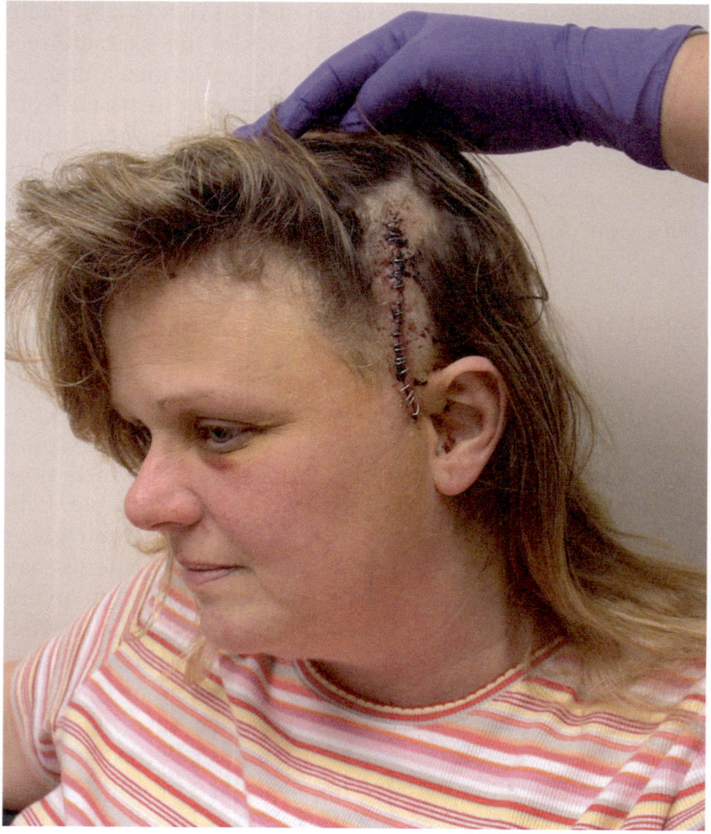

FIGURE 10.9 Postoperative incision with staples in patient a with recent left-sided bypass

hormones, especially those with estrogen, increase stroke risk. Barrier methods are safest for birth control. Pregnancy is well tolerated after recovery from moyamoya surgery, and no special precautions are necessary, such as cesarean delivery. We recommend continuation of aspirin therapy during pregnancy. Patients should avoid wearing tight eyeglasses or anything that compresses the skin in front of the ear where

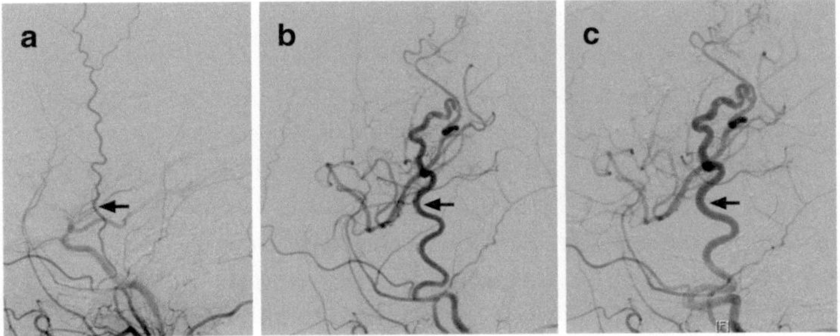

FIGURE 10.10 Superficial temporal (scalp) artery (STA) angiogram. (**a**) Preoperative parietal branch of the ECA (*arrow*). (**b**) Postoperative 6 month angiogram shows enlarging bypass filling the brain through the STA (*arrow*). (**c**) Three year postoperative angiogram shows further enlargement of the STA bypass filling brain (*arrow*)

the donor artery is close to the surface. Otherwise, helmets and headgear are fine. Maintaining adequate hydration is important, and we recommend drinking 2 l of non-caffeinated liquids daily. Caffeinated drinks are fine, but should not be counted as part of the 2 l. Patients should refrain from donating blood to prevent loss of overall blood volume. Maintaining a healthy blood pressure (110–140/70–90) is recommended, and we always advise our patients to contact us before starting any medication for blood pressure reduction.

Long Term Outcome

We recommend that patients return for follow-up at 6 months, and 3, 10 and 20 years after surgery (Fig. 10.10). Our overall patient clinical and radiological outcomes are excellent. The long-term incidence of stroke after bypass is exceptionally low, and TIAs are significantly reduced [8]. Unilateral patients are at risk for progressing to the other side, and we therefore recommend a yearly MRI or CT angiogram to monitor for progression [14].

Summary

Increasing awareness over the past 20 years of moyamoya symptoms and diagnosis has improved access to care for patients. Excellent surgical options are available to treat moyamoya, and surgery has been shown to be superior to medical therapy alone at preventing strokes, with excellent overall long term outcomes and minimal interruptions in lifestyle. We strongly advocate increased patient education and awareness of moyamoya, and encourage patients to be actively engaged with the treatment team to optimize long-term outcomes.

Funding Sources Josef Huber Family Moyamoya Fund, Stanley and Alexis Shin, Reddy Lee Moyamoya Fund, William Randolph Hearst Foundation, Bernard and Ronni Lacroute, Russell and Elizabeth Siegelman.

References

1. Abla AA, et al. Surgical outcomes for moyamoya angiopathy at barrow neurological institute with comparison of adult indirect encephaloduroarteriosynangiosis bypass, adult direct superficial temporal artery-to-middle cerebral artery bypass, and pediatric bypass: 154 revascularization surgeries in 140 affected hemispheres. Neurosurgery.2013;73(3):430–9.doi:10.1227/NEU.0000000000000017.
2. Achrol AS, et al. Pathophysiology and genetic factors in moyamoya disease. Neurosurg Focus. 2009;26(4):E4. doi:10.3171/2009.1.FOCUS08302.
3. Achrol AS, et al. In reply. The genetics of moyamoya disease: recent insights into the pathogenesis of the disease. Neurosurgery. 2013;72(2):E321–322. doi:10.1227/NEU.0b013e31827bc1c1.
4. Calviere L, et al. Executive dysfunction in adults with moyamoya disease is associated with increased diffusion in frontal white matter. J Neurol Neurosurg Psychiatry. 2012;83(6):591–3. doi:10.1136/jnnp-2011-301388.
5. Chiu D, et al. Clinical features of moyamoya disease in the United States. Stroke. 1998;29(7):1347–51.
6. Choi JU, et al. Natural history of moyamoya disease: comparison of activity of daily living in surgery and non surgery groups. Clin Neurol Neurosurg. 1997;99 Suppl 2:S11–18.

7. Dorfman LJ, et al. Moyamoya disease can masquerade as multiple sclerosis. Neurologist. 2012;18(6):398–403. doi:10.1097/NRL.0b013e31826a99a1.

8. Guzman R, et al. Clinical outcome after 450 revascularization procedures for moyamoya disease. Clinical article. J Neurosurg. 2009;111(5):927–35. doi:10.3171/2009.4.JNS081649.

9. Guzman R, et al. Direct bypass techniques for the treatment of pediatric moyamoya disease. Neurosurg Clin N Am. 2010;21(3): 565–73. doi:10.1016/j.nec.2010.03.013.

10. Hallemeier CL, et al. Clinical features and outcome in North American adults with moyamoya phenomenon. Stroke. 2006;37(6):1490–6. doi:10.1161/01.STR.0000221787.70503.ca.

11. Kamada F, et al. A genome-wide association study identifies RNF213 as the first Moyamoya disease gene. J Hum Genet. 2011;56(1):34–40. doi:10.1038/jhg.2010.132. jhg2010132 [pii].

12. Karzmark P, et al. Neurocognitive impairment in adults with moyamoya disease without stroke. Neurosurgery. 2012;70(3):634–8. doi:10.1227/NEU.0b013e3182320d1a.

13. Karzmark P, et al. Effect of moyamoya disease on neuropsychological functioning in adults. Neurosurgery. 2008;62(5):1048–51. doi:10.1227/01.neu.0000325866.29634.4c; discussion 1051–1042.

14. Kelly ME, et al. Progression of unilateral moyamoya disease: a clinical series. Cerebrovasc Dis. 2006;22(2–3):109–15. doi:10.1159/000093238.

15. Khan N, et al. Sex differences in clinical presentation and treatment outcomes in Moyamoya disease. Neurosurgery. 2012;71(3):587–93. doi:10.1227/NEU.0b013e3182600b3c; discussion 593.

16. Khan N, et al. Failure of primary percutaneous angioplasty and stenting in the prevention of ischemia in Moyamoya angiopathy. Cerebrovasc Dis. 2011;31(2):147–53. doi:10.1159/000320253.

17. Kim SK, et al. Pediatric moyamoya disease: an analysis of 410 consecutive cases. Ann Neurol. 2010;68(1):92–101. doi:10.1002/ana.21981.

18. Kuroda S, et al. Radiological findings, clinical course, and outcome in asymptomatic moyamoya disease: results of multicenter survey in Japan. Stroke. 2007;38(5):1430–5. doi:10.1161/STROKEAHA.106.478297. doi: STROKEAHA.106.478297 [pii].

19. Kuroda S, et al. Incidence and clinical features of disease progression in adult moyamoya disease. Stroke. 2005;36(10): 2148–53. doi:10.1161/01.STR.0000182256.32489.99.

20. Kurokawa T, et al. Prognosis of occlusive disease of the circle of Willis (moyamoya disease) in children. Pediatr Neurol. 1985;1(5): 274–7. 0887-8994(85)90027-X [pii].

21. Miskinyte S, et al. Loss of BRCC3 deubiquitinating enzyme leads to abnormal angiogenesis and is associated with syndromic moyamoya. Am J Hum Genet. 2011;88(6):718–28. doi:10.1016/j.ajhg.2011.04.017. S0002-9297(11)00158-3 [pii].
22. Navarro R, et al. Less-invasive pedicled omental-cranial transposition in pediatric patients with moyamoya disease and failed prior revascularization. Neurosurgery. 2013. doi:10.1227/NEU.0000000000000119.
23. Pandey P, et al. Patients with moyamoya disease presenting with movement disorder. J Neurosurg Pediatr. 2010;6(6):559–66. doi:10.3171/2010.9.PEDS10192.
24. Scott RM, et al. Moyamoya disease and moyamoya syndrome. N Engl J Med. 2009;360(12):1226–37. doi:10.1056/NEJMra0804622.
25. Scott RM, et al. Long-term outcome in children with moyamoya syndrome after cranial revascularization by pial synangiosis. J Neurosurg. 2004;100(2 Suppl Pediatrics):142–9. doi:10.3171/ped.2004.100.2.0142.
26. Smith ER, et al. Moyamoya: epidemiology, presentation, and diagnosis. Neurosurg Clin N Am. 2010;21(3):543–51. doi:10.1016/j.nec.2010.03.007.
27. Starke RM, et al. Moyamoya disorder in the United States. Neurosurgery. 2012;71(1):93–9. doi:10.1227/NEU.0b013e318253ab8e.
28. Starke RM, et al. Clinical features, surgical treatment, and long-term outcome in adult patients with moyamoya disease. Clinical article. J Neurosurg. 2009;111(5):936–42. doi:10.3171/2009.3.JNS08837.
29. Suzuki J, et al. Cerebrovascular "moyamoya" disease. Disease showing abnormal net-like vessels in base of brain. Arch Neurol. 1969;20(3):288–99.
30. Takeuchi K, et al. Hypoplasia of the bilateral internal carotid arteries. Brain Nerve. 1957;9:37–43.
31. Zach V, et al. Headache associated with moyamoya disease: a case story and literature review. J Headache Pain. 2010;11(1):79–82. doi:10.1007/s10194-009-0181-8.

Chapter 11
Medical Management of a Stroke

Mary Guhwe, Kelly Blessing, Susan Chioffi, and Carmelo Graffagnino

What Is a Stroke?

The two major types of stroke are classified as ischemic stroke or hemorrhagic stroke. An ischemic stroke happens when the blood flow to the brain is stopped by narrowing or blockage of an artery by a blood clot or by cholesterol. As a result, the brain does not get blood or oxygen and some parts of the brain

M. Guhwe, RN, MSN, FNP-BC, SCRN (✉)
Department of Neurology, Duke University Medical Center,
Erwin Road, Durham, NC 27710, USA
e-mail: Mary.guhwe@duke.edu

K. Blessing, FNP
Department of Neurology, Duke University Medical Center,
2900 Bryan Research Building Research Drive,
Durham, NC 27710, USA
e-mail: Kelly.blessing@duke.edu

S. Chioffi, RN, MSN, ACNP-BC
Department of Neurology, Duke University Medical Center,
Erwin Road, Durham, NC 27710, USA
e-mail: Susan.chioffi@duke.edu

C. Graffagnino, MD
Department of Neurology, Duke University Medical Center,
2900 Bryan Research Building Research Drive, Durham,
NC 27710, USA
e-mail: Carmelo.graffagnino@duke.edu

A. Agrawal, G. Britz (eds.), *Emergency Approaches to Neurosurgical Conditions*, DOI 10.1007/978-3-319-10693-9_11,
© Springer International Publishing Switzerland 2015

die [1]. A hemorrhagic stroke happens when bleeding occurs in the brain. This can happen because of bleeding from a blood vessel which breaks or due to a recent ischemic stroke [1].

Signs and Symptoms of Stroke

A stroke is a medical emergency. Once symptoms of stroke are noted, call 911 without delay. This is because it activates specific steps related to the treatment of stroke for Emergency Medical Services personnel (EMS) and for the emergency room. Signs of a stroke include:

Sudden face drooping
Sudden weakness on one side of the body
Sudden numbness on one side of the body
Sudden change in vision or vision loss
Sudden confusion
Sudden speech or language difficulty (slurred speech, difficulty understanding or difficulty reading and writing)
Sudden onset of headache from unknown cause
New sudden coordination difficulties
Sudden new difficulties with balance or walking

Most stroke symptoms are sudden and obvious. However at times they can be subtle and progress over hours to days. Even if symptoms go away, still call 911 as this may be a warning of a bigger problem if left untreated. Figure 11.1 shows the key events in the treatment and recovery of stroke.

Treatment of Ischemic (Clotting) Stroke

In the event of an ischemic stroke, the first goal is to get blood flowing to the affected area of the brain quickly to prevent brain cells from dying. This is why calling 911 at the first sign of symptoms is especially important for possible treatment with alteplace (tPA). This medication dissolves clots that block arteries within the brain. The quicker tPA is given, the more effective it is [2]. Studies have shown that

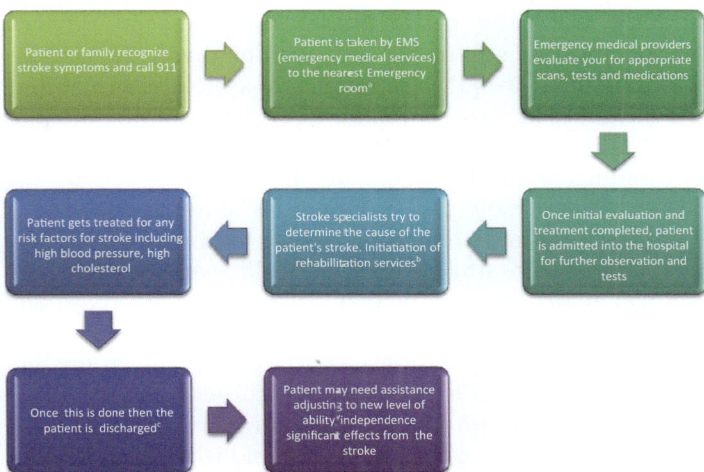

FIGURE 11.1 Summary of evaluation and treatment of stroke. [a]Patients and family should call 911 and let EMS transport patient to the emergency room as this triggers certain protocols and treatment guidelines that allow timely management and treatment. [b]Determining the cause of a stroke is important to prevent future strokes or reduce risk of future strokes. However sometimes a definite cause is not found even with a complete workup. [c]Patients may be discharged home, to sub-acute rehabilitation facility or to acute rehabilitation facility depending on their level of symptoms and ability to participate in the different therapies

patients that receive tPA often have a better recovery compared to those that did not receive treatment with tPA. However, tPA does not come without risk. There is a 6 % chance of bleeding into the area of stroke associated with this treatment [2]. The important thing to remember is that patients receiving tPA have the same risk of dying compared to those that did not receive tPA. Thus, despite the bleeding risk, receiving tPA does not increase your risk of dying when compared to not receiving tPA. Another treatment option is an endovascular procedure. This is when doctors with advanced training try removing the blood clot directly from the blood vessel using special devices. Researchers are still trying to determine the best situations for this procedure [3]. Once initial treatment is completed, the medical team will continue to closely monitor the person. In the first few days after a large stroke, there is a risk of swelling in the brain due to the injury caused by the stroke. The person can become sick enough to need a breathing tube and breathing machine because they become too sleepy to breathe properly. Should swelling occur, the medical team can use medicines to try to decrease the amount of swelling. In severe cases, when the patient meets strict criteria, an operation called a hemicraniectomy can be done. When this is done, a neurosurgeon takes part of the person's skull off giving the brain more space to swell outwards. The piece of skull is saved and will be put back in place several months later. In the mean time, the person's head is protected by a special helmet until the skull can be put back on [6].

Immediately after the stroke, the stroke patient will not be allowed to eat or drink until their swallowing is tested. A stroke often affects the swallowing muscles which could result in food going into the lungs and causing pneumonia which would prolong recovery or in some cases could result in death [3]. Stroke patients with swallowing problems will work with Speech Therapists to learn to swallow safely.

The stroke patient's blood pressure will be left high for several days after the stroke to maximize blood flow to the affected area of the brain. This prevents death of brain cells around the area of the stroke [3]. Their heart will be checked for an irregular heart rhythm called atrial fibrillation. This heart rhythm poses significant risk of stroke and the patient may need to be on lifelong blood thinners if found to have this rhythm. There will be other scans and blood tests ordered depending on medical and family history.

Treatment of Hemorrhagic (Bleeding) Stroke

In a hemorrhagic stroke, a blood vessel in the head breaks and blood leaks out into the brain and sometimes the spinal fluid. There is very little room in a person's head for anything extra such as blood which is no longer contained in a blood vessel so this kind of stroke often makes a person very ill immediately and they have to go to an Intensive Care Unit [4]. With this kind of stroke people may immediately become unconscious and require a breathing tube and ventilator (breathing machine) while being treated. The blood which has leaked out can cause the pressure inside the person's head to become very high causing brain damage and even death. Special monitors are often used to monitor the pressure inside the brain. Specific medicines can be used to try to control the high pressure. Sometimes the person has to be sedated(made very sleepy) or kept very cold to allow the brain time to heal from the effects of the high pressure [4, 5]. The blood from bleeding into the brain is mixed in with brain tissue so surgery to try to remove the clot is usually not helpful. Just like with ischemic strokes, sometimes an operation called a hemicraniectomy might be done to relieve the high pressure by giving the brain room to swell outwards and have time to heal [7]. Sometimes people may have seizures from the blood irritating the brain. They will get medicine to treat the seizures and prevent future seizures. Seizures can affect recovery from the initial stroke and change how someone functions in their day to day activities. The person needs to be extra careful about activities in which they or people around them could be seriously hurt if they were to have a seizure. In the United States as a safety measure, after a person has a seizure, he or she is not allowed to drive until a certain amount of time has passed in which they do not have seizures. This time frame varies from state to state [4]. Sometimes, the bleeding that happens is very small and while someone becomes sick enough to come to the hospital, they do not become sick enough to go to the ICU. They still have to stay in the hospital while their medical team finds out why the bleeding occurred. Often it is because a person's blood pressure is too high and needs to be controlled better. If the person was taking any kind of blood thinner, this will be stopped to give the brain time to heal. When they leave the hospital, they will usually be asked not to take any over-the-counter pain medication besides acetaminophen. Other widely available pain medicines can increase the risk of bleeding. When the person is seen in clinic for follow up by a neurologist, they may need to get follow up brain scans. Sometimes bleeding in the brain is caused by a tumor or a malformed vessel that was not seen initially because the blood in the brain made it hard to see. It takes several weeks for the blood to resolve and allow anything that might be there to be seen properly [5].

Recovery from Stroke

Stroke recovery and rehabilitation often starts as soon as the survivor is treated for the stroke. Depending on the location and amount of brain tissue affected by the stroke, the ability of a person to recover and benefit from rehabilitation varies. After the acute phase of either kind of stroke, the brain and body may be able to recover some, if not all, of the function that was lost. This time period of recovery may last days, months, and even years. Generally, the process of recovery is most rapid in the first few weeks and this often sets the rate for further improvement. Rehabilitation is begun as soon as possible, often while the patient is still in the hospital. Rehabilitation focuses both on maintaining the person's current abilities as well as the regaining of functions affected by the stroke. Stroke rehabilitation involves the patient, family, caregivers, and a variety of healthcare specialists. As every patient and stroke is different, the healthcare specialists needed to assist in the patient's rehabilitation may vary as outlined in Table 11.1. The number of specialties involved in the process may be overwhelming to

TABLE 11.1 Members of the medical team and rehabilitation team

Physicians/ advanced practice providers	These include primary care providers that are essential in the management of stroke risk factors such as blood pressure, diabetes and cholesterol. Neurologists are doctors who specialize in problems of the brain and nerves. Neurosurgeons are doctors who specialize in surgery of the brain, spine, and nerves
Physical therapist	Specializes in physical activities such as balance and walking as well as strengthening and maintaining mobility in the body. If required, they help patients learn to properly use a walker or cane
Occupational therapist	Works to help regain function in affected limbs or help the person learn new ways of doing things so that the patient may regain the ability to perform daily tasks such as feeding, dressing, bathing. They may also help evaluate safety needs such as special equipment needed for the home
Speech therapist and pathologist	They evaluate the person's ability to swallow and recommend the types of foods that are safe while working with the person to improve impaired swallowing abilities. Help patients to improve language skills such as speech, reading and writing. Also they may assist with learning to manage memory and thinking problems
Social worker	Help to identify resources needed for persons in the community. These may include assistance with financial decisions, living arrangements, and transportation
Dieticians	Assist with identifying healthy diets that will give the patient the most optimal nutrition
Psychologist	May be needed to assess thinking skills and behavioral needs after strokes

both patients and their families. It is important to understand their roles as they will be working with the patient and families through recovery and rehabilitation. In some cases, the patient can be discharged to their home with outpatient therapy, done through a community center or hospital. For patients with debilities that make travel difficult, home therapy may be available. In other cases, a patient may leave the hospital to go to an inpatient rehabilitation facility for several weeks before they are able to return home. It is important to remember that some patients are too sick or disabled after a stroke to be able to participate in rehabilitative therapies. In these cases, therapy may be deferred. Occasionally, when a person's disabilities require a large amount of nursing care, the best option for the patient and their family is discharge from the hospital to a skilled nursing facility or nursing home.

Complications of Strokes

Depending on the parts of the brain affected by the patient's stroke, the stroke survivor may experience ongoing effects that limit their ability to bathe, dress, eat, walk, and toilet without assistance. Table 11.2 provides a brief summary of common terms used to describe problems that stroke survivors may encounter. Problems with communication may also occur as a result of strokes. Communication problems may involve trouble saying the right words or being able to write or read. Often the person knows what they want to communicate but simply "cannot get the words out". This can be very frustrating for the person as well as their loved ones. In can also involve slurring or unclear speech. The person may say the right words but the speech can be hard to understand. Sometimes the muscles used to swallow correctly are affected by strokes, making choking a very real concern. If a person has difficulty swallowing, he or she may not be able to eat a normal diet. Sometimes the person may require thickened fluids and soft foods so that they do not

TABLE 11.2 Common problems after stroke

Aphasia	A disturbance in which ability to comprehend, formulate, read, or write is impaired
Dysarthria	The inability to clearly speak due to muscle weakness of the face, mouth, or respiratory system
Dysphagia	Difficulty swallowing
Paresis	Weakness of the muscles used to move a body part
Paralysis	The inability to move a body part
Incontinence	The involuntary loss or urine or feces

inhale food into their lungs. If the swallowing difficulties are severe, it may require special feeding tubes so that the person is able to have adequate nutrition while they recover. Some strokes cause odd sensations, pain, and numbness that can be frustrating for patients and their caregivers. The patient and caregivers can work with the patient's provider to see if medication can help with these kinds of discomfort. Urinary problems such as incontinence (leaking or accidents) may be related to weakness or damage to certain areas of the brain. Fortunately, many of the effects of strokes may continue to improve with time and intensive rehabilitative therapy. The stroke survivor may have also have problems with memory, attention, and depression. Depression after a stroke can be serious, even in people who have never had depression before. Family members, friends, and caregivers can assist in watching for symptoms of depression. Depression can interfere with a person's ability to adequately participate in their rehabilitation program. Medications and specialized therapy can often assist with reducing depression. Also, patients may find that physical intimacy and sexual relations have been impacted after a stroke. This may be due to both physical and emotional changes. Physical changes may be due to the stroke itself as well as medications. Emotionally, patients may have a fear of causing another stroke or may feel less desire because of depression and stress. Most survivors can return to active healthy intimacy as soon as they desire. However, the person's doctor can provide guidance in returning to sexual intimacy if there is a concern.

Preventing Another Stroke

Controlling hypertension (high blood pressure) is very important after a stroke. High blood pressure damages arteries and the organs, including the brain, supplied by those arteries. Blood pressure medicines reduce the high pressure and assist in keeping the arteries from getting more damage. Patients with strokes are often started on blood pressure medication or they may have their previous medications changed. Blood pressure medicines work in different ways and often patients will need more than one medication to get the best results. Caregivers and family members are encouraged to ask the patient's doctors or nurses what the patient's "goal" blood pressure is and help the person with monitoring their blood pressure at home. This lets their doctors know how well the medicines are working and if more adjustments need to be made. People with diabetes or high blood sugars are more likely to have recurrent strokes [8]. High blood sugars change the lining of the blood vessels, causing them to be more likely to become blocked. Various members of the health care team can work with the patient and family to achieve proper control of blood sugars through a combination of diet, medicine, and exercise. High cholesterol is also a risk factor for more strokes and is often treated with medication. Sometimes people only learn they have high cholesterol when they have a stroke and will need to start medicine. Sometimes people were already on cholesterol lowering medicines and will have the doses or medicines changed because of a stroke. After an ischemic (blocked artery) stroke, the goal will be to get the cholesterol levels much lower than those set for most people [9]. The treatment of cholesterol most often involves medications known as "statins". These potent cholesterol medications have been shown to improve outcomes in certain stroke survivors [10]. For survivors of ischemic stroke, their medications will often include aspirin or medications like aspirin, known as antiplatelet agents. Antiplatelet agents have been shown to reduce the risk of ischemic stroke [11]. These medications keep parts of the blood from sticking together inside the arteries. Blood thinners or anticoagulation is different from antiplatelet agents. These medications are most frequently used for patients who have had abnormal heart rhythms that cause blood clots to form in the heart. Patients with bleeding types of stroke may be advised to never take antiplatelet agents or anticoagulants as they may interfere with the ability to seal off ruptured blood vessels. Stopping smoking is one of the most effective ways to reduce a person's risk for stroke. Smoking is a strong risk factor for ischemic stroke [12–14]. There are many resources available to assist patients to quit even if they have been unsuccessful in their attempts before. The patient's doctor and health care team can assist in locating good resources to make the process easier.

Maintaining healthy weight, healthy diet, and exercise as well as reduction in heavy alcohol intake play a vital role in reduction of stroke risk but also in general health.

Resources

National Stroke Association
9707 East Easter Lane
Suite B
Centennial, CO 80112-3747
info@stroke.org
http://www.stroke.org
Tel: 303-649-9299 800-STROKES (787–6537)
American Stroke Association: A Division of American Heart Association
7272 Greenville Avenue
Dallas, TX 75231-4596
strokeassociation@heart.org

148   M. Guhwe et al.

http://www.strokeassociation.org
Tel: 1-888-4 STROKE (478–7653)
Brain Aneurysm Foundation
269 Hanover Street, Building 3
Hanover, MA 02339
office@bafound.org
http://www.bafound.org
Tel: 781-826-5556 888-BRAIN02 (272–4602)
National Aphasia Association
350 Seventh Ave.
Suite 902
New York, NY 10001
naa@aphasia.org
http://www.aphasia.org
Tel: 212-267-2814 800-922-4NAA (4622)

References

1. Caplan LR. Caplan's stroke: a clinical approach. 4th ed. Philadelphia: Saunders Elsevier; 2009.
2. The National Institute of Neurological Disorders and Stroke rt-PA Stroke Study Group. Tissue plasminogen activator for acute ischemic stroke. N Engl J Med. 1995;333(24):1581–7.
3. Jauch EC, Saver JL, Adams HP, Bruno A, Connors JJ, Demaerschalk BM, et al. On behalf of the American Heart Association Stroke Council, Council on Cardiovascular Nursing, Council on Peripheral Vascular Disease, and Council on Clinical Cardiology Guidelines for the Early Management of Patients With Acute Ischemic Stroke. A guideline for healthcare professionals from the American Heart Association/American Stroke Association. Stroke. 2013;44:870–947.
4. Hickey JV. The clinical practice of neurological and neurosurgical nursing. 6th ed. Philadelphia: Wolters Kluwer/Lippincott Williams & Wilkins; 2009.
5. Baird MS, Bethel S. Manual of critical care nursing: nursing interventions and collaborative management. 6th ed. St. Louis: Elsevier Mosby; 2011.
6. Vahedi K, Vicaut E, Mateo J, Kurtz A, Orabi M, Guichard J-P, Boutron C, Couvreur G, Rouanet F, Touze E, Guillon B, Carpentier A, Yelnik A, Georg B, Payen D, Bousser M-G. A

sequential design, multicenter, randomized, controlled trial of early decompressive craniectomy in malignant middle cerebral artery infarction (DECIMAL trial). Stroke. 2007;38:2506–17.

7. Fung C, Murek M, Z'Graggen WJ, et al. Decompressive hemicraniectomy in patients with supratentorial intracerebral hemorrhage. Stroke. 2012;43(12):3207–11.

8. Callahan A, Amerenco P, Goldstein L, Sillesen H, Messig M, Samsa G, Altafullah I, Ledbetter L, MacLeod M, Scott R, Hennerici M, Zivin J, Welch M. Risk of stroke and cardiovascular events after ischemic stroke or transient ischemic attack in patients with type 2 diabetes or metabolic syndrome: secondary analysis of the stroke prevention by Aggressive Reduction in Cholesterol Levels (SPARCL) trial. Arch Neurol. 2011;68(10):1245–51.

9. Furie K, Kasner S, Adams R, Albers G, Busch R, Fagan S, Halperin J, Claiborne Johnston S, Katzan I, Kernan W, Mitchell P, Ovbiagele B, Schwamm L, Wassertheil-Smoller S, Turan T, Wentworth D, American Heart Association/American Stroke Association. Guidelines of the prevention of stroke in patients with stroke or transient ischemic attack. Stroke. 2011;42:227–76. doi:10.1161/STR.0b013e3181f7d043. Published online before print. October 21, 2010.

10. Amarenco P, Beavente O, Goldstein L, Callahan A, Sillesen H, Hennerici M, Gilbert S, Rudolph A, Simunovic L, Zivin JA, Welch M, on behalf of the SPARCL Investigators. Results of the stroke prevention by Aggressive Reduction in Cholesterol Level (SPARCL) trial by stroke subtypes. Stroke. 2009;40:1409.

11. Antithrombotic Trialist' Collaboration. Collaborative meta-analysis of randomized trials of anti-platelet therapy for the prevention of death myocardial infarction, and stroke in high risk patients [published correction appears in BMJ 2002; 324:1]. BMJ. 2002;324(7329):71–86.

12. Shinton R, Beevers G. Meta-analysis of relation between cigarette smoking and stroke. BMJ. 1989;298(6676):789–94.

13. Gill J, Shipley M, Tsementzi S, Hornby R, Gill S, Hitchcock E, Beevers D. Cigarette smoking. A risk factor for hemorrhagic and nonhemorrhagic stroke. Arch Intern Med. 1989;149(9):2053–7.

14. Wolf P, D'Agostino R, Kannel W, Bonita R, Belanger A. Cigarette smoking as a risk factor for stroke: the Framingham Study. JAMA. 1988;259:1025–9.

Chapter 12
Neuro-Interventional Management of a Stroke

Jan Vargas, Alejandro M. Spiotta, Raymond Turner, Imran Chaudry, and Aquilla S. Turk

Incidence of Stroke

Each year almost 800,000 people suffer a new or recurrent stroke. Of these, 87 % ischemic strokes, due to a blockage of vessels going into the brain. About 55,000 more women suffer from strokes a year, and in general women are more likely to have a stroke [1]. Ischemic strokes are most commonly caused by either a rupture of an atherosclerotic plaque, or by a blood clot that forms in another part of the body (most commonly the heart) and travels into the blood vessels of the brain.

J. Vargas, MD (✉) • A.S. Turk, DO
Department of Radiology and Radiological Sciences,
Medical University of South Carolina, Charleston, SC, USA
e-mail: jav8@musc.edu; turk@musc.edu

A.M. Spiotta, MD
Department of Neurosurgery, Medical University of South
Carolina, Charleston, SC 29425, USA

R. Turner, MD
Department of Neurosurgery, Medical University of South Carolina,
Charleston, SC, USA

I. Chaudry, MD
Department of Radiology, Medical University of South Carolina,
Charleston, SC, USA

A. Agrawal, G. Britz (eds.), *Emergency Approaches to Neurosurgical Conditions*, DOI 10.1007/978-3-319-10693-9_12,
© Springer International Publishing Switzerland 2015

Symptoms of Stroke

Ischemic strokes can occur suddenly and can lead to devastating consequences. Timely recognition and response is critical. The American Stroke Association has created the F.A.S.T. mnemonic to aid the diagnosis of an ischemic stroke and to facilitate delivery of patients to the hospital. F.A.S.T stands for "(F)acial droop, (A)rm weakness, (S)peech difficulty, (T)ime to call 911."The first three letters represent some of the most common symptoms of an ischemic stroke, and stress the urgency of quickly transporting patients to the nearest hospital for evaluation and possible transfer to a stroke center.

How Will My Family Member Be Evaluated for My Stroke?

Once at a stroke center, the patient is evaluated by stroke neurologists. If warranted, the next step in work up will usually include specialized imaging, such as computed tomography (CT) of the head with or without perfusion. If there is no evidence of a bleed found on the head CT, and if there is a strong suspicion for an ischemic stroke, the patient will be evaluated for treatment.

What Treatment Options Are There for a Stroke?

Currently, the only FDA approved treatment for ischemic strokes is the administration of intravenous tissue plasminogen activator (IV tPA), known more colloquially as a "clot buster." Current guidelines state that IV tPA must be administered within 4.5 h after the onset of symptoms [2]. Patients who are candidates for receiving IV tPA include patients who are more than 18 years of age and have a clinical diagnosis of an ischemic stroke. Some patients are not eligible for IV tPA, such as those with active or recent bleeding (including intracranial hemorrhage), major surgery or trauma in the previous 2 weeks, GI or urinary bleeding within 3 weeks, or a systolic blood pressure of greater than 185 mmHg or a diastolic blood pressure of more than 110 mmHg.

For those patients who are ineligible for IV tPA, one option includes intra arterial (IA) treatment. In order to qualify for this type of treatment, a patient must have a significant amount of brain tissue that has not been irreversibly damaged by the interruption of blood flow. This area of salvageable brain is termed the "ischemic penumbra," and represents brain cells that have been momentarily stunned by the interruption of oxygen.

Intra arterial (IA) therapy takes place in an angiography suite, which is similar to a surgical operating room but is equipped with specialized machines to provide the necessary imaging to perform these procedures safely. The procedure can be done with the patient either asleep under general anesthesia as they would for a surgical operation or with some relaxing medication. At some centers, the preference is to perform these procedures with the patient awake but comfortable, so that the treating physicians can evaluate how the patient is doing and if the stroke symptoms are responding to the therapy, in other words if the patient is now able to move his or her arms or legs when before they were unable to. In some instances, the results can be very dramatic with the patient becoming completely normal on the table at the conclusion of the procedure.

IA therapy consists of puncturing a large artery, usually the femoral artery, and then placing catheters and wires to access the blood vessels supplying oxygen to the brain, similar to a heart catheterization for heart attacks. Navigation of the catheters takes place under direct visualization with fluoroscopy, which is a form of radiation like an xray. Gaining access to the cerebral blood vessels provides a platform for a variety of treatment strategies to restore blood flow to the brain. There are risks to such a procedure, the most common being post procedural bleeding from the catheter insertion site in the groin, to damage to blood vessel walls (also known as a dissection), to more serious complications such as blood vessel perforation and subsequent bleeding in the head, as well as worsening stroke.

Beginning in the late 1990s with the administration of intra arterial prourokinase, another "clot buster," the field of intra arterial therapy has rapidly evolved. The first generation of devices were aspiration catheters with maceration wires that were positioned next to intra arterial clots and used to macerate and restore blood flow. These systems were replaced by newer devices, called "stent retrievers," which have been shown in studies to be effective at restoring blood flow [3–5]. Stent retrievers differ from their predecessors in that they engage the clot and the physician removes it from within the blood vessel. More recently, physicians have begun directly aspirating blood clots, which allows for restoration of blood flow to occur in minutes [6]. While it may seem that these different technologies have replaced older methods, in practice many physicians use combinations of these techniques to restore blood flow to the brain. In some cases direct aspiration will be attempted as a first line treatment, but if that fails some practitioners may employ stent retrievers. Concomitantly, intra arterial tPA can be given at the same time for smaller showered clots that are not amenable to mechanical clot removal. While intra arterial methods of mechanically disrupting or removing the clot hold a lot of promise, they are as of yet unproven in a scientific study, although several studies are ongoing at this time.

What Can I Expect from My Family Member Following a Stroke?

The importance of quickly treating patients with acute ischemic stroke has been borne out in several studies, demonstrating the fact that the faster a patient's blood flow to the brain is restored, the faster they will recover [7, 8]. In about 50 % of cases, physicians can restore blood flow to the brain in a matter of minutes. It is important to realize that ischemic strokes can be devastating, and it may take up to a year of intensive physical therapy and rehabilitation for a patient to recovery. Additionally, while many patients can make significant progress, ischemic strokes can be debilitating and many people will not fully recover. The goal of quickly restoring blood flow to the brain is to provide patients with the best chance at a good recovery.

References

1. Go AS, Mozaffarian D, Roger VL, Benjamin EJ, Berry JD, Blaha MJ, et al. Heart disease and stroke statistics–2014 update: a report from the American Heart Association. Circulation. 2014;129(3):e28–292. PubMed PMID: 24352519.
2. Hacke W, Kaste M, Bluhmki E, Brozman M, Davalos A, Guidetti D, et al. Thrombolysis with alteplase 3 to 4.5 hours after acute ischemic stroke. N Engl J Med. 2008;359(13):1317–29.
3. Levy EI, Ecker RD, Horowitz MB, Gupta R, Hanel RA, Sauvageau E, et al. Stent-assisted intracranial recanalization for acute stroke: early results. Neurosurgery. 2006;58(3):458–63; discussion –463. PubMed PMID: 16528185.
4. Nogueira RG, Lutsep HL, Gupta R, Jovin TG, Albers GW, Walker GA, et al. Trevo versus Merci retrievers for thrombectomy revascularisation of large vessel occlusions in acute ischaemic stroke (TREVO 2): a randomised trial. Lancet. 2012;380(9849):1231–40. PubMed PMID: 22932714.
5. Saver JL, Jahan R, Levy EI, Jovin TG, Baxter B, Nogueira RG, et al. Solitaire flow restoration device versus the Merci Retriever in patients with acute ischaemic stroke (SWIFT): a randomised, parallel-group, non-inferiority trial. Lancet. 2012;380(9849):1241–9. PubMed PMID: 22932715.
6. Turk AS, Spiotta A, Frei D, Mocco J, Baxter B, Fiorella D, et al. Initial clinical experience with the ADAPT technique: a direct aspiration first pass technique for stroke thrombectomy. J Neurointervent Surg. 2014;6(3):231–7. PubMed PMID: 23624315.
7. Rha JH, Saver JL. The impact of recanalization on ischemic stroke outcome: a meta-analysis. Stroke. 2007;38(3):967–73. PubMed PMID: 17272772.
8. Sun CH, Nogueira RG, Glenn BA, Connelly K, Zimmermann S, Anda K, et al. "Picture to puncture": a novel time metric to enhance outcomes in patients transferred for endovascular reperfusion in acute ischemic stroke. Circulation. 2013;127(10):1139–48. PubMed PMID: 23393011.

Chapter 13
Symptoms and Signs to Look for After a Spinal Cord Injury

Graham H. Creasey

At the Scene of an Accident

Look for loss of movement and ask about loss of feeling in the arms and legs, which may indicate a spinal cord injury (SCI). This loss of function may be at any level from the shoulders down. Loss of movement or feeling in the arms or hands suggests an injury in the neck; loss of movement or feeling from the chest down suggests an injury in the back. Pain in the spine may or may not be present.

If there is any suspicion of a spinal cord injury, even if there is no loss of movement or feeling, treat the person as if they have a spinal cord injury until proved otherwise.

The neck and spine should be kept still while waiting for ambulance personnel, who should have special collars to immobilize the neck. The person should be transported with their spine immobilized on a firm stretcher or backboard to an acute hospital capable of treating major trauma.

G.H. Creasey, MB, ChB, FRCSEd
Department of Neurosurgery,
Stanford University School of Medicine,
VA Palo Alto Health Care System,
3801 Miranda Ave, Palo Alto, CA 94304, USA
e-mail: gcreasey@stanford.edu

A. Agrawal, G. Britz (eds.), *Emergency Approaches to Neurosurgical Conditions*, DOI 10.1007/978-3-319-10693-9_13,
© Springer International Publishing Switzerland 2015

At an Acute Hospital

The person will be assessed first in an emergency room to determine whether they have any other injuries. They will then be admitted to the hospital and may have an operation to stabilize their spine. Their breathing and blood pressure will also be stabilized. Their bladder will probably be drained by a catheter initially, and their bowels should be emptied regularly to avoid constipation. It is important for them to be turned or moved every couple of hours to avoid prolonged pressure on the skin over bony areas.

After being stabilized medical and surgically it is important to go through comprehensive inpatient rehabilitation to learn the skills of living with a SCI and to improve the prospects of a good quality of life. Look for a SCI Unit or Center specializing in this type of rehabilitation as described below. Lists of such centers are available at the websites below [1, 2].

At a Comprehensive Rehabilitation Center

Inpatient SCI rehabilitation requires a specialized team of physicians, nurses, occupational and physical therapists, psychologists, social workers and other staff, with appropriate experience and equipment. They provide specialized training in learning to live with loss of movement or feeling and managing the many other consequences of spinal cord injury such as altered bladder and bowel function, and restoring sexual function such as erection and the ability to have children. They provide information about control of blood pressure and temperature, pain, and spasticity that can produce involuntary contractions of muscle and jerking of the limbs. They also provide specialized training in learning to prevent complications such as pneumonia, urine infection and pressure ulcers. They also assist with emotional adjustment of the person injured and their family, and social adaptations such as housing, driving, education and employment.

During and after inpatient rehabilitation, look for a team of health care providers who can work together to provide both specialist care for the effects of SCI and primary care for other general health issues. The way to maximize quality of life after SCI is to have such a team that can offer comprehensive care and regular follow-up for life. Also look for role models who are living well with a spinal cord injury and who can be mentors and friends.

At Home

Maintaining health and maximizing function and quality of life requires consistent attention to prevent complications of SCI, such as the following.

Skin Breakdown

If a person does not have sensation they do not realize when the circulation has been cut off from a part of their skin on which they have been lying or sitting for too long. This can result in severe damage to the skin and underlying tissues, which can be followed by infection of these tissues and large pressure ulcers. At least twice a day look for red marks on the skin, particularly over bony areas such as the tailbone, hip bones and buttocks. If such red marks are found, avoid lying or sitting on that area of skin until the marks have faded.

Urine Infection

The bladder often does not empty properly after SCI. The urine in the bladder can become infected and this infection can spread to the kidneys and the bloodstream and be serious. If a person has impaired sensation, they may not realize this. Symptoms and signs of urine infection include feeling generally unwell, urine that smells different or is cloudy, and a raised temperature or pulse rate.

Sometimes the infection spreads down to the testes, and this can damage fertility. Initially this infection may have no symptoms but signs include a swollen testis, which may also be warm.

If a person has a catheter in the bladder, this can become blocked. If this happens, the pressure in the bladder can rise, causing a dangerous rise in blood pressure called autonomic dysreflexia. Symptoms and signs of this include a pounding headache, often with a low pulse rate, flushing of the face, and a stuffy nose. It is urgent to relieve the pressure in the bladder by unblocking or changing the catheter. This rise in blood pressure can also be caused by distended bowel or rectum, or any other conditions that would be painful in a person with sensation. Temporary relief may be gained by sitting up, and medications to lower the blood pressure can be made available for first aid.

Pneumonia

People with SCI find it difficult to cough and breathe deeply, particularly if the injury is in their upper spine, and are prone to pneumonia. They may be aware of increased secretions in their chest and breathlessness, in addition to other signs of infection such as a temperature and rapid pulse. It is important to get prompt medical attention, probably with antibiotics and respiratory therapy.

Constipation

This may initially be evident as feeling generally unwell or bloated. A combination of high fiber diet, laxatives, and suppositories or enemas can be used to prevent or treat it.

Fractures

After SCI the bones below the level of the injury become weaker because of disuse. Fractures of the leg can occur with minor injuries, and may not be noticed for some time because of the lack of sensation. Signs of such a fracture include swelling around the knee or ankle, abnormal mobility or position of the limb, and sometimes increased spasticity. In time the skin may become bruised or red and may break down because of pressure from the broken bones. It is important to immobilize the limb with plenty of padding to protect the skin.

Further Spinal Cord Damage

Loss of feeling and movement may improve slightly during the first year or two after a SCI, but then usually remains stable. If there is further loss after this time, or new symptoms such as pain or tingling, it is important to have this investigated medically to search for any new problems.

At Other Hospitals or Emergency Rooms

If you become ill and need treatment at a hospital or emergency room that is not familiar with spinal cord injury, the staff may need to be reminded of some of the complications of SCI, such as autonomic dysreflexia, as well as the importance of regular turning to prevent pressure ulcers, and regular emptying of the bladder and bowels. It can be useful to put them in touch with a specialized Spinal Cord Injury Center for consultation or a second opinion [3, 4].

When Evaluating Research

Spinal cord injury has historically caused permanent paralysis, but research is being carried out into ways of restoring function using technology and, perhaps in the future, with stem cells. In evaluating this research it is important to look for features of high quality ethical clinical trials using the principles described by the International Collaboration on Repair Discoveries [5].

When Traveling

Look for seating that will not cause pressure ulcers and relieve pressure regularly. Inform airlines or travel agencies of any special needs, including transport of wheelchairs, and allow extra time for boarding and transfers. Spinal cord injury need not prevent you from traveling widely and having an adventurous life! [6]

References

1. Spinal Cord Injury Model System Information Network. https://www.uab.edu/medicine/sci/uab-scims-information.
2. Spinal Cord Injuries and Disorders, US Department of Veterans Affairs. www.sci.va.gov/index.asp.
3. Spinal Cord Injury Model Systems. http://www.msktc.org/sci/model-system-centers.
4. VA Spinal Cord Injury and Disorders Centers. http://www.sci.va.gov/SCI_Centers.asp.
5. International Collaboration on Repair Discoveries. www.icord.org/research/iccp-clinical-trials-information/.
6. Walsh A, editor. Able to travel: true stories by and for people with disabilities. London: Rough Guides Ltd; 1994.

Chapter 14
Evaluation of Spinal Alignment

G. Alexander West

The human spine is divided into three major segments: cervical, thoracic, and lumbosacral regions. Each spinal segment is made of vertebra and discs. The cervical segment has 7, thoracic 12 and lumbar 5 segments. The sacrum has 5 segments which are usually fused together with the lumbar and sacrum often considered together. The vertebral segments contain the spinal cord, surrounding the spinal canal as bony elements to protect the spinal cord within the canal. Each segment is separated by discs that act as a cushion between each bony segment. The skull rests on the top cervical vertebra, C1 or the Atlas. The spinal nerves exit each level of the spine from the spinal cord from the cervical region all the way to the sacrum. The solid spinal cord usually ends at L1 level, with the nerves continuing within the spinal canal to the scarum.

G.A. West, MD, PhD
Department of Neurosurgery,
Houston Methodist Hospital, Houston, TX, USA
e-mail: gawest@houstonmethodist.org

A. Agrawal, G. Britz (eds.), *Emergency Approaches to Neurosurgical Conditions*, DOI 10.1007/978-3-319-10693-9_14,
© Springer International Publishing Switzerland 2015

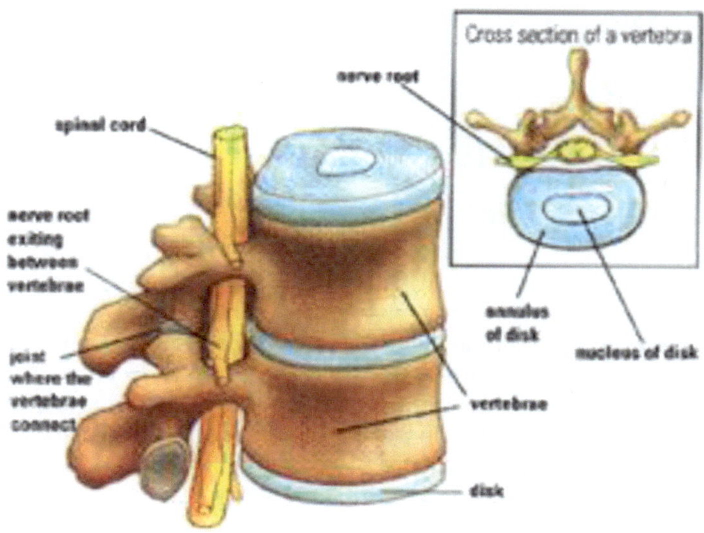

Side view of two vertebrae

In the erect spine with the person standing the spine has a specific alignment. From the front, the coronal plane, the skull and spine should be straight. From the side, sagittal plane, the spine has three main curves, with the shape of two "S's". The top S curve in the cervical spine is lordotic. The thoracic spine and sacrum are lordotic. The lumbar spine is kyphotic. With normal posture and alignment the curves should balance each other out such that the head is in alignment with the pelvis, "normal sagittal" alignment exists. Spinal alignment is important for humans for walking and standing. Efficient use of energy in walking depends on good spinal alignment. In addition, when there is normal alignment there is usually no pain with upright posture and the muscles around the spine are less likely to fatigue. When the head is aligned over the pelvis no extra energy is needed in walking and the spine is considered "balanced".

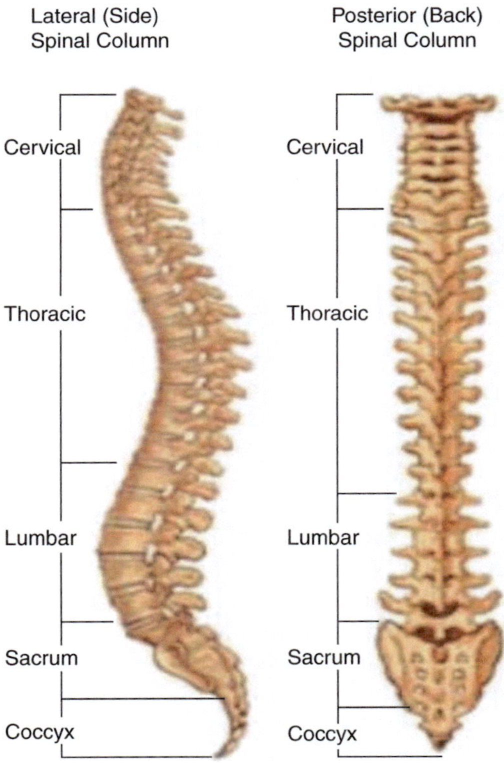

When there is malalignment of the spine often this may reflect problems. Acute change in alignment most often results from trauma. Traumatic injuries can cause minor injury to the muscle and soft tissue around the spine and may cause mild changes in alignment. Most of these minor changes in alignment can be managed conservatively with medication for pain or muscle spasms, application of heat/cold, physical therapy and other modalities. Moderate or severe injuries to the spine may cause injuries to the ligaments which connect to the vertebra to each other or fractures of the bony elements of the spine. The injury may cause a direct injury to the spinal cord or nerve roots resulting in neurological deficits. If there is a change in alignment that creates instability of the spine, either an external brace or surgery is needed to stabilize the spine.

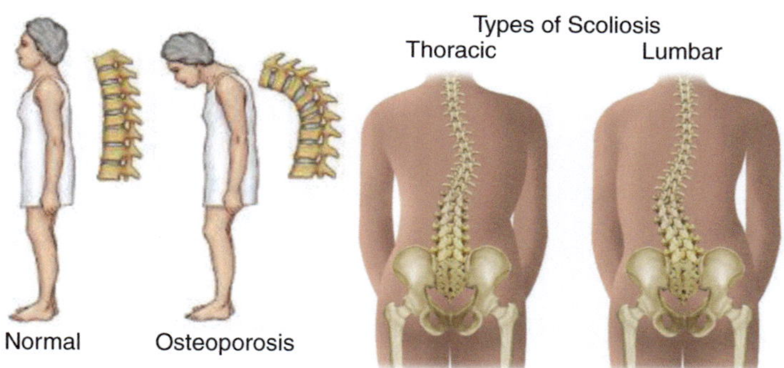

In addition to trauma which usually can cause an acute change in spinal alignment, other conditions can cause changes in a very gradual fashion. As we age the disc between the vertebra degenerate, losing water. Sometimes with degenerative disc there can be a significant loss of height in the thoracic spine that may result in kyphosis which may be mild or sometimes progress enough to need treatment. Other conditions may cause a change in the coronal alignment, developing a curve when looking at the spine in the front to back view is called scoliosis. Scoliosis is common and can be asymptomatic in may cases when the curve is not severe. Often scoliosis is balanced, with a "compensatory curve". When scoliosis is progressive it may cause symptoms that require surgery.

Changes in the sagittal alignment can also reflect progressive degenerative disease or a pathological problem. When the spine angles forward, it is called kyphosis, or forward bending of the spine. With kyphosis it may result in the head positioned forward of the pelvis and sagittal imbalance. If kyphosis progresses and there is sagittal imbalance this can result in several issues for patients that require treatment with either bracing or surgical treatment. Surgery can be effective is correcting alignment in the spine, either scoliosis or kyphosis when there is both scoliosis and kyphosis. The malalignment can involve on segments of the spine, cervical, thoracic or lumbar or combinations of the different levels of the spine. The greater number of vertebra, the more complex can be the problem and the surgery to correct it.

Making the diagnosis of abnormal spinal alignment is very important in patients. In the setting of trauma, diagnosing instability is critical for proper management of the patient after an acute injury. If the patient has normal neurological function but an injury to the ligaments or vertebra, stabilizing the spine is critical to prevent secondary injury to the spinal cord and nerves. After an injury most patients are placed in a C-collar and on a backboard to temporarily hold the spine in alignment. Usually CT scans of the spine, MRI or plain x-rays are done to assess the patient's spine. The imaging studies usually can assess the injury and allow proper management decisions on treating the patient.

For degenerative disease imaging studies are also used to make a diagnosis of spinal alignment. Usually MRI and standing x-rays are done to assess the patient's condition. A CT scan may be needed as well since the CT can give more detailed images of the bony anatomy. MRI's can give images of the spinal cord and nerves but like the CT scan is obtained with patient lying down. Upright x-rays can show both the coronal views, front to back view, and sagittal, lateral, view. X-rays can also be obtained with the patient bending forward, back and sideways which can show if there is abnormal movement of the spine. Thus, imaging studies are tools used to assess the patient's problem and along with the patient's symptoms and history determine appropriate treatment. In the acute setting when there is a traumatic injury of the spine, usually a CT scan is sufficient to evaluate the spine and establish whether instability is present. MRI may be needed to better evaluate whether the spinal cord is injured or there is possible ligament injury which can cause instability.

In summary, evaluation of spinal alignment is very important in assessing acute spinal injury as well degenerative disease. With an acute injury, it is critical to establish whether there is malalignment and instability of the spine. Treatment is dictated by the type and amount of injury. In degenerative disease, abnormal alignment of the spine is usually a slowly progressive problem that can lead to pain, neurological deficits and other symptoms. In some cases malalignment in degenerative disease is chronic and maybe stable and not cause symptoms or require treatment. Imaging, including plain x-rays, CT scan and MRI are important studies that allow assessment of spinal alignment. Treatment recommendations for patients should include awareness of the spinal alignment as well as other factors in order to provide good treatment.

Chapter 15
Herniated Discs of the Spine

Brandon D. Liebelt and J. Bob Blacklock

Anatomy

Discs are named based upon their adjacent vertebrae. For instance, the L4-L5 disc is the disc that lies between the fourth lumbar and fifth lumbar vertebrae. They are up to 3/8 in. thick and 1 and 5/8 in. wide in the lumbar spine, but are smaller in the cervical and thoracic regions [1]. The disc is composed of an outer layer, the annulus fibrosis, and an inner region, the nucleus pulposus. The annulus fibrosis is a leather-like outer covering of the disc. The nucleus pulposus is the gelatin like material within the disc which aids in cushioning and distributing forces placed on the spine. If a tear occurs in the annulus fibrosis and nucleus pulposus protrudes through the tear, a herniation of the disc occurs.

B.D. Liebelt, MD (✉) • J.B. Blacklock, MD
Department of Neurosurgery,
Methodist Neurological Institute, Houston, TX, USA
e-mail: bdliebelt@tmhs.org; bblacklock@tmhs.org

A. Agrawal, G. Britz (eds.), *Emergency Approaches to Neurosurgical Conditions*, DOI 10.1007/978-3-319-10693-9_15,
© Springer International Publishing Switzerland 2015

Cervical Spine

The cervical spine is composed of seven vertebrae, and eight paired cervical nerves exit at each level. The cervical spinal cord occupies the spinal canal just behind the vertebrae and discs. Herniated discs in this region can cause compression of not only the nerve roots, but also of the spinal cord itself. Symptoms of herniated cervical discs can cause cervical radiculopathy, from compression of nerve roots, or myelopathy, from compression of the spinal cord.

Cervical Radiculopathy

Radiculopathy refers to damage or irritation of a specific nerve root with symptoms occurring in one or both arms. A disc herniation compressing a nerve root can be the cause. The two most commonly involved levels are C5-C6 and C6-C7, with C6-7 occurring in nearly 70 % of cases [2].

Cervical Myelopathy

Cervical myelopathy occurs when there is compression of the spinal cord. This can result from herniated discs, bone spurs, or from traumatic fractures with dislocation of the spine. Symptoms of myelopathy include hand weakness, gait instability, and balance issues.

Treatment

Conservative treatment options include the use of nonsteroidal anti-inflammatory medications, oral steroids, epidural steroid injections, physical therapy, and activity modifications. However, surgery may be needed when conservative measures have failed to solve the symptoms. Surgical options include anterior cervical discectomy and fusion or posterior approaches (laminectomy or foraminotomy). The anterior approach involves an incision in the front of the neck and removal of the intervertebral disc at the involved levels. A fusion is performed in this procedure to stabilize the spine since the disc has been removed. A graft is placed between the adjacent vertebrae and a metal plate and screws are used to connect the two vertebrae. Posterior approaches involve an incision in the back of the neck and removal of either the entire lamina (laminectomy) to decompress the spinal cord or removal of only a small portion of bone to decompress individual nerve roots (foraminotomy). Each procedure has its own advantages and disadvantages depending on the individual patient's pathology. These procedures can often be performed as an outpatient operation.

Thoracic Spine

The thoracic spine is composed of 12 vertebrae and 12 spinal nerves. Each thoracic vertebrae has a corresponding rib attached. This confers additional stability and less mobility to the thoracic spine and is the reason disc herniations occur much less frequently in this region. Thoracic disc herniations comprise only 0.25 % of all herniated discs [3]. Herniated discs usually occur at levels at or below T8 [4]. The first seven ribs are directly attached to the sternum and therefore is the more stable portion of the thoracic spine. Herniated thoracic discs most commonly cause radiculopathy but can also cause myelopathy.

Thoracic radiculopathy is typically experienced as pain radiating from the mid back around the ribcage. Sensory changes, such as numbness and parasthesias (pins and needles sensation) can also occur. Muscle weakness is typically not present as the thoracic nerves do not innervate muscles of the arms or legs. Symptoms from myelopathy in the thoracic spine are similar to the symptoms from cervical myelopathy but affect only the legs.

Treatment

Indications for surgical treatment of herniated thoracic discs include refractory pain or progressive myelopathy. Surgery for herniated thoracic discs is more complicated than in the cervical or lumbar spine. Thoracic herniated discs are calcified in 65 % of cases that present for surgery [4]. This makes them less mobile and more difficult to remove. For this reason a direct midline approach through the back is typically not used as the spinal cord would lie directly between the surgeon and the herniated disc. Lateral approaches through the side are typically used and often require partial removal of a rib in order to access the disc. While more invasive, this angle will allow the easiest access to the herniated disc with the least risk of damage to the spinal cord.

Lumbar Spine

The lumbar spine is composed of five vertebrae and five corresponding lumbar spinal nerves exit at each level. The first sacral nerve root traverses the L5-S1 disc space and can be compressed by a herniated disc at this level. Disc herniations in this region can result in symptoms of radiculopathy, neurogenic pseudoclaudication, or cauda equina syndrome depending on the size and location of the herniation.

Lumbar Radiculopathy

Lumbar radiculopathy is the most common form of radiculopathy. Disc herniations occur in this region most frequently as a result of the added stress and weight the lumbar spine is exposed to. Sciatica is radiculopathy that involves either the L5 or S1 nerve roots and is felt as pain that radiates down the back or outside of the leg down to the foot. L5 and S1 radiculopathy are the most common forms, accounting for around 90–95 % of lumbar radiculopathy. L3 and L4 radiculopathy are typically felt in the front of the thigh. L2 radiculopathy is felt in the groin, and L1 radiculopathy is felt just above the groin. In addition to pain, numbness and weakness in the leg can also be experienced.

Neurogenic Pseudoclaudication

Neurogenic pseudoclaudication is the result of lumbar stenosis (narrowing of the spinal canal). Disc herniations can contribute to lumbar stenosis but there are typically multiple factors involved. Other contributing factors include thickened ligaments around the spine and arthritic changes of the vertebrae. The symptoms of neurogenic pseudoclaudication are experienced as leg fatigue, heaviness, and weakness when walking. This is usually relieved by sitting down, resting, or leaning forward.

Cauda Equina Syndrome

The cauda equina is the collection of nerve roots within the spinal canal below the end of the spinal cord. A very large disc herniation which compresses multiple nerve roots can lead to cauda equina syndrome. Symptoms may include urinary retention or incontinence, bowel incontinence, numbness in the genital region, leg weakness or paralysis, low back pain, and leg pain.

Treatment

Conservative options are similar to the nonsurgical treatments in the cervical spine. Indications for surgery are refractory pain, progressive weakness, and cauda equina syndrome. A discectomy is performed to remove the herniated disc and relieve the pressure on the nerve root(s). The patient is placed in the facedown, or prone, position for surgery. A midline incision is made in the lower back and the lamina of the involved level is exposed. A small laminotomy, or opening in the lamina, is made to allow enough room to access the intervertebral disc. An operating microscope is often used to allow for better visualization. The herniated disc fragment is then removed, leaving the remainder of the disc in its anatomic position between the vertebral bodies. Many times this can be accomplished with a minimally invasive, outpatient procedure.

References

1. Raj PP. Intervertebral disc: anatomy-physiology-pathophysiology-treatment. Pain Pract. 2008;8(1):18–44.
2. Mayfield FH. Cervical spondylosis: a comparison of the anterior and posterior approaches. Clin Neurosurg. 1965;13:181–8.
3. El-Kalliny M, Tew Jr JM, van Loveren H, Dunsker S. Surgical approaches to thoracic disc herniations. Acta Neurochir (Wien). 1991;111(1–2):22–32.
4. Stillerman CB, Chen TC, Couldwell WT, Zhang W, Weiss MH. Experience in the surgical management of 82 symptomatic herniated thoracic discs and review of the literature. J Neurosurg. 1998;88(4):623–33.

Chapter 16
Spinal Fusion

Paul J. Holman, Blake Staub, and Matthew McLaurin

Indications

Fusion surgery is indicated in a variety spine conditions including degeneration, deformity, tumors, and trauma. Degenerative conditions are the most common indication for fusion surgery. Examples include degenerative disc disease, spondylolisthesis (misaligned bones), and facet syndrome (pain due to arthritis in spinal joints).

Surgical Techniques

The specific techniques used by surgeons to achieve a successful spinal fusion have evolved significantly over the past several years. Newer implants, minimally (MIS) invasive surgery, and new bone grafting materials all continue to be refined to give more consistent results and a quicker recovery than in the past.

P.J. Holman, MD (✉) • B. Staub, MD
Department of Neurosurgery, Methodist Neurological Institute, 6560 Fannin, Suite 944, Houston, TX 77030, USA
e-mail: pjholman@tmhs.org; bnstaub@houstonmethodist.org

M. McLaurin
Louisiana State University, Baton Rouge, LA 70803, USA

A. Agrawal, G. Britz (eds.), *Emergency Approaches to Neurosurgical Conditions*, DOI 10.1007/978-3-319-10693-9_16,
© Springer International Publishing Switzerland 2015

There are two parts of a fusion: <u>spinal hardware</u> and <u>bone graft</u>. The fusion ultimately occurs because bone grafts help the patient's own bone to build a bridge linking the vertebrae together. For many years the gold standard for bone graft was bone harvested from the hipbone. Because this graft is harvested from the patient's own body, it is referred to as *autograft*. Unfortunately, as many as 15 % of patients noted chronic hip pain at the site of bone removal. Many alternatives to hip bone grafting have been developed to avoid this potential complication. The most common alternative is *allograft* – human bone taken from a cadaver. Newer allograft products include cadaver bone that is specifically engineered to include a higher concentration of adult stem cells – cells known to encourage new bone formation. The cadaver bone is tested and processed to minimize the chance for disease transmission or rejection by the recipient.

Two more recently popularized alternative bone-grafting materials are bone morphogenic proteins (BMPs) and bone marrow aspirate (BMA). BMA is taken by inserting a small needle into the hip during surgery. Only the liquid bone marrow is removed providing a rich source of bone growth promoting substances. BMPs are genetically engineered proteins that stimulate bone formation. BMP is a very powerful bone growth tool, but as with any new technology, it can occasionally create unwanted side effects. It is important to know that most spinal surgeons use BMPs in an "off-label" manner. This means that they are used in areas of the spine not approved by the Food and Drug Administration (FDA). Using medications off-label is quite common in many fields of medicine and it is the responsibility of the surgeon to discuss the expected outcomes and possible complications with the patient.

The second major component of a typical spinal fusion surgery is the spinal hardware – "rods and screws". For bone to heal it must be fixated in one spot. Spine surgeons use specialized tools to fix the spine in place around the bone graft to allow a bony bridge to form between the two bones to be fused. No, the hardware will not set off the metal detector in the airport. And no, it does not ever need to come out unless there is a complication.

Preoperative Considerations

Prior to any type of spinal fusion a patient should undergo a full medical work-up to rule out or treat any potential underlying medical issue.

In addition, it is imperative that there is good communication between the patient and the surgeon in regard to both the risks and benefits of the surgical procedure. No surgery will be successful unless the patient and the surgeon expect the same result.

Recovery from a spinal fusion does not happen overnight. Patients must consider their social situation before undergoing any surgical procedure. Large fusion operations can keep a person out of work for months at a time and can take a significant physical and emotional toll on families.

Postoperative Considerations

After the surgery has been completed, patients will be taken to the post-anesthesia recovery unit to begin recuperating. Here they are monitored for a safe recovery from anesthesia with frequent assessment of vital signs and administration of pain medication. Fusions done through a "posterior" approach involve incisions in the rear of the neck or lower spine and typically cause the most postoperative pain because of the manipulation of the spinal muscles. Many surgeons choose to initially treat the patient's pain with a "PCA", or Patient Controlled Anesthesia system where safe doses of narcotics are delivered into the bloodstream only when the patient chooses to push a button. This helps patients to actively participate in their recovery. Additional medications administered after surgery include muscle relaxers and sometimes anti-inflammatory agents. The PCA is generally discontinued within 1–2 days after surgery as the patient's pain becomes easier to control with oral medications. Anterior cervical fusions require less muscle manipulation and are generally much less painful.

After surgery it is normal to have pain at the site of the incision. In addition, it is not uncommon to have some residual leg or arm pain. Generally, this is due to swelling around the nerves or manipulation of the nerves during surgery. This routinely improves within the first 1–2 post-operative days and should not be a major cause for concern unless the symptoms are severe or progressive. Any weakness or numbness that was present before surgery will likely be present immediately after the surgery. Muscle weakness can also be new or slightly worse postoperatively and should be assessed by the surgeon. Nerve damage can take up to 12–15 months for a maximum recovery. Some degree of weakness can be permanent if preoperative deficits are severe. The exact degree of nerve recovery is unpredictable. As a general rule, the longer the symptoms exist prior to surgery, the less likely they are to fully recover.

In the days to weeks following surgery, patients are given specific activity guidelines. Although a modest amount of walking is encouraged to prevent complications, more is not necessarily better. A restriction on how much weight to lift will be set by the surgeon to avoid stress on the muscles, joints, and nerves that are in the healing process. Patients who undergo lumbar procedures should avoid bending, twisting, and leaning forward at the waist. Depending on the area of the spine fused and surgeon preference, the surgeon may recommend use of a postoperative brace.

Most fusion surgeries still require a variable period of inpatient hospitalization. Cervical fusions performed thru the front of the neck are typically the least painful and patients are usually discharged the morning after surgery. Fusions performed through the back muscles typically require inpatient recovery. Although minimally invasive approaches aim to minimize muscle trauma, patients can still expect to be hospitalized 2–3 days. Complex fusions of multiple vertebral levels require bigger incisions and longer hospitalization, particularly if surgery is "staged" –performed on more than 1 day to minimize the risk associated with very long surgeries.

A physical therapist may be consulted in the hospital to help in your recuperation. The patient's pain level should improve each day after surgery although some day-to-day variation in pain is not uncommon. In general, a patient is ready for discharge once they can manage surgical pain without intravenous narcotics, urinate, address constipation, and walk safely with minimal assistance (or with a walker or cane). Patients that live alone or who do not have a family member that is capable of providing enough support may benefit from an additional week or longer in a rehabilitation unit.

The need for outpatient, postoperative, physical therapy can be helpful to strengthen specific muscles that were weak prior to surgery due to nerve damage. Therapy can also improve the collection of "core" muscles that support the global function and alignment of the spine.

Determining Success

The success of a spinal fusion operation can be assessed by both clinical and radiographic markers. The criteria for radiographic success include formation of a solid bridge of bone between the vertebrae included in the operation. This can take 3–12 months to occur. This is typically confirmed by spinal x-rays and a CT scan. A failure of fusion is referred to as a "pseudoarthrosis" and can be identified by persistent motion between the vertebral bones, loosening or breakage of the hardware, and absence of new bone formation on postoperative radiographs.

Clinical success for spinal fusion is determined by the degree of improvement in both the symptoms affecting the patient prior to surgery and in the improvement in quality of life and function.

Conclusion

Spinal fusion surgery is a safe and effective medical treatment for a variety of spine conditions. New technology emerges every year to make these procedures safer and less painful.

A successful fusion requires not only the skill and knowledge of the surgeon but also patient participation in the recovery.

Chapter 17
Spinal Cord Tumors

Robert E. Isaacs and Vijay Agarwal

Introduction

A spine tumor is an abnormal mass of tissue from, or surrounding, the spine. The cells of the tumor multiply in an uncontrolled fashion. Tumors of the spine can involve either the spinal cord or the vertebral bodies, the stacked bones in the back that protect the spinal cord. Included in this category are tumors of the layer covering the spinal cord, or the meninges, and the cauda equina (latin for "horse's tail"), or the loose bundle of nerves as they progress downward from the tip of the spinal cord. They can occur in the cervical region (neck), the thoracic region (middle back), or the lumbosacral region (lower back). In addition, they are classified according to whether they are in the front (anterior) or back (posterior) of the spine. These types of tumors account for 2–4 % of all tumors of the central nervous system [1]. Even though the spine is part of the central nervous system that includes the brain, tumors in the spine are unique and have their own diagnostic and treatment characteristics. However, just as in the brain, tumors in the spine can be benign or

R.E. Isaacs, MD (✉) • V. Agarwal, MD
Division of Neurological Surgery, Department of Surgery,
Duke University Medical Center, Durham, NC, USA
e-mail: Robert.isaacs@duke.edu; vjagarwal@gmail.com

A. Agrawal, G. Britz (eds.), *Emergency Approaches to Neurosurgical Conditions*, DOI 10.1007/978-3-319-10693-9_17,
© Springer International Publishing Switzerland 2015

malignant (cancerous). The three categories that spinal cord tumors are classified in are the following: (1) intramedullary, arising from the actual spinal cord itself, (2) intradural-extramedullary, arising from the dura (the layer covering the spinal cord) but outside the actual spinal cord, and (3) extra-dural, arising most often from the vertebral bodies. Extramedullary tumors comprise the vast majority of tumors (~90 %). Metastatic tumors from elsewhere in the body can occur in any of these three categories, but the overwhelming majority are extradural.

Symptoms

Tumors in the spine cause symptoms because of the impor-tant and abundant nerves and nerve pathways that course through the area. These nerves relay information to and from peripheral parts of the body and the brain, and affect movement, sensation, balance, and pain. One of the most common symptoms is pain that causes the patient to awaken from sleep; it is a gnawing and unremitting sensa-tion, and may be able to indicate where the tumor actually is [2]. However, pain can truly originate anywhere along the long nerve pathways. Other symptoms include problems with sensation, weakness of muscles, decreased sensitivity to pain, heat, and cold, loss of bowel or bladder function, or paralysis of various degrees. Difficulty with basic functions that use these muscles, such as walking and lifting objects, is often times affected. This is particularly dangerous because it can lead to falls. Interestingly, these symptoms may start on one side of the body, but as both sides of the spinal cord become affected bilateral symptoms result. Using broad categories, symptoms can be divided into pain or neurologic deficits. Pain can be persistent or intermit-tent, and is often not relieved by rest or medication. Neurologic deficits are caused by nerve root compression and/or spinal cord compression, and frequently include altered gait. Classically, tumors in the cervical (neck) region may cause numbness or weakness in the arms or legs, while thoracic or lumbosacral tumors may cause numbness or weakness in the chest or leg area. Difficulty walking can occur with tumors anywhere along this axis. As back pain is common, and because there are many causes for it, knowing when to see a doctor is difficult to determine. Since early detection and treatment of these tumors is very important, a person would be advised to see their doctor if they experience the following symptoms: persistent or worsening pain, pain that is not related to specific activities, pain that is worse at night (especially when attempting to sleep), and a history of cancer [3]. The spine is a common place for other cancers to spread to, or metastasize, such as prostate cancer, breast cancer, and lung cancer [4, 5]. Urgent medical attention should be given to worsening muscle weakness or numbness or problems with bowel or bladder function. For this reason, a very complete physical examination by a doctor is required to check for probable sites of where the tumor is, checking baseline preoperative function, and the check the status of gait.

Risk Factors

Most spinal tumors have no known cause. Rarely, they can be caused by exposure to certain cancer causing agents or chemicals. Lymphoma may occur in patients whose immune system is compromised. There are two known genetic diseases that can lead to spinal cord tumors. Neurofibromatosis Type 2 causes noncancerous growths to develop on or near nerves. Some people with this disease may develop tumors in the spinal cord. Von Hippel-Lindau disease is a rare disorder of noncancerous blood vessel tumors known as hemangioblastomas in the brain, retina, and spinal cord. A prior history of cancer, of any type, can put a person at risk for spread to the spine. However, the cancers with the highest rates of spread to the spine include breast, lung, prostate, and multiple myeloma.

Laboratory Findings

Most often, laboratory findings in patients with spinal cord tumors do not show specific abnormalities. However, there are some specific types of tumors that are exceptions to this. These would include a high protein content in the blood in multiple myeloma, an increase in the enzyme acid phosphatase in prostate cancer metastasis, an increase in the catecholamine metabolite vanillylmandelic acid (VMA) in the urine in neuroblastoma, an increase in the enzyme alkaline phosphatase in osteosarcoma, and increased blood counts in lymphoma.

Intramedullary Tumors

Tumors in this category arise from the spinal cord itself (Fig. 17.1). As mentioned, these tumors only make up ~10 % of the total number. The majority of tumors in this location are "gliomas". They are called this because under a microscope they resemble a type of cell called the glial cell. These cells form the outer coat of neurons in the nervous system, and provide support and protection. The types of glial tumors

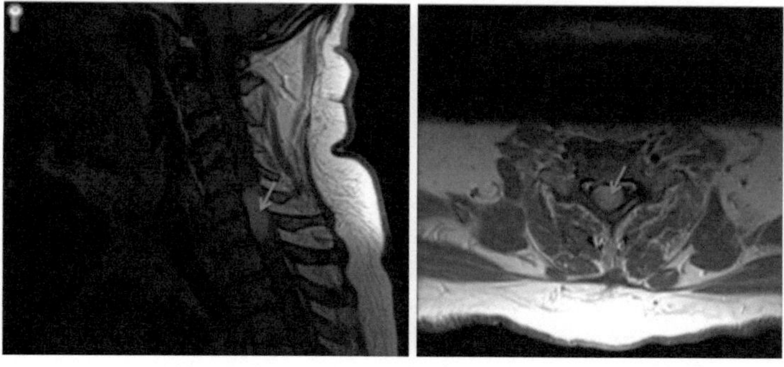

FIGURE 17.1 MRI scan showing intramedullary spinal cord tumor (*blue arrows*) on side view (sagittal, *left image*) and top view (axial, *right image*) of spine

common here are ependymomas, astrocytomas, and oligodendrogliomas. Ependymomas are the most common in adults, with usual age between 30 and 40 years. Ependymal tumors are split into four major groups: ependymoma, myxopapillary ependymoma (mostly in the lumbosacral area), subependymoma, and anaplastic ependymoma. Further subdivisions of ependymomas are cellular (most common), papillary, clear cell, and tancytic types. The reason intramedullary tumors are generally so uncommon, is because the amount of glial tissue is significantly less in the spinal cord than the brain.

Intradural Extramedullary Tumors

Tumors in this category arise from, or under, the outer layer of the spinal cord (dura), but external to the actual spinal cord (Fig. 17.2). Meningiomas and nerve sheath tumors (from the covering of the nerves) can develop in this compartment. Nerve sheath tumors include schwannomas and neurofibromas. Spinal meningiomas are most commonly in the thoracic spine, and grow very slow. Often times, they also have high calcium content [6]. Schwannomas and neurofibromas are benign nerve sheath tumors, but neurofibromas have the potential to become cancerous.

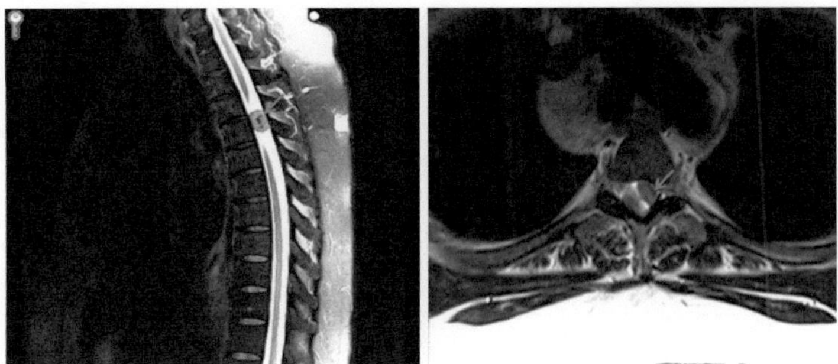

FIGURE 17.2 MRI scan showing intradural extramedullary spinal cord tumor (*blue arrows*) on side view (sagittal, *left image*) and top view (axial, *right image*) of spine

Extradural Tumors

Tumors in this category most often arise from the vertebral bodies (Fig. 17.3). As discussed, metastasis can occur anywhere in the spine, but will most often arise here, and are the most common extradural spine tumor. The most common metastasis in this area include prostate cancer, breast cancer, and lung cancer. This location is also home to several uncommon primary tumors. Tumors found here include: chordomas (rare bone tumors), sarcomas (usually in younger patients), lymphoma, plasmacytomas and multiple myeloma, and eosinophilic granuloma (Langerhans cell histiocytosis). Benign (nonmalignant) tumors in this category include: osteoid osteomas (found in long bones, <2 cm in size), osteoblastomas (>2 cm in size), osteochondromas (which has both bone and cartilage), chondroblastomas (arises from immature cartilage), giant-cell tumors, vertebral hemangiomas (composed of thing-walled blood vessels, and rarely cause symptoms), and aneurysmal bone cysts.

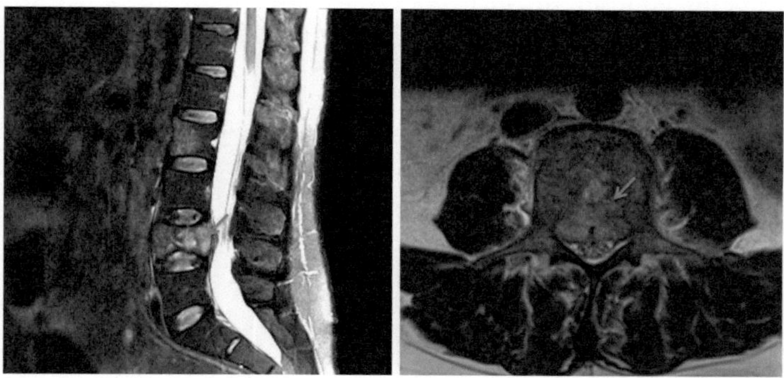

FIGURE 17.3 MRI scan showing extradural spinal cord tumor (*blue arrows*) on side view (sagittal, *left image*) and top view (axial, *right image*) of spine

Imaging

An x-ray can show the basic bony structure of the spine, and the outline of the joints. It is often a good way to eliminate causes other than tumors for back pain, such as fractures. However, x-rays are not a very reliable way to diagnose spine tumors. Computed Tomography (CT scan) is used to create an image of the spine to show the general shape and size of the spinal canal and the structures around it. A CT scan is often the best modality to visualize bony structures. Magnetic resonance imaging (MRI) uses magnetics to produce 3-D images of the spine. An MRI can show the spinal cord, nerve roots, spinal degeneration, and a higher level of details than a CT scan. It is the best imaging to obtain to diagnose a spinal cord tumor.

Management

Treatment for these spine tumors depends on what the preliminary diagnosis is. Often, after confirmation of tumor with an MRI, it is necessary to obtain a small piece to test, known as a biopsy. This can be done through a very small hole to obtain a small piece of tissue to determine benign versus malignant, and the exact type. The treatment your doctor will choose depends on multiple factors, such as the location and specific type of the tumor. Sometimes, surgery can be curative. Other times, options may include a combination of surgery and radiation therapy. Chemotherapy is much less commonly used.

References

1. Chamberlain MC, Tredway TL. Adult primary intradural spinal cord tumors: a review. Curr Neurol Neurosci Rep. 2011;11(3): 320–8.

2. Welch WC, Jacobs GB. Surgery for metastatic spinal disease. J Neurooncol. 1995;23(2):163–70.
3. Welch WC, et al. Systemic malignancy presenting as neck and shoulder pain. Arch Phys Med Rehabil. 1994;75(8):918–20.
4. Black P. Spinal metastasis: current status and recommended guidelines for management. Neurosurgery. 1979;5(6):726–46.
5. Posner JB. Neurologic complications of cancer, Contemporary neurology series. Philadelphia: Oxford University Press; 1995.
6. Lee JW, et al. CT and MRI findings of calcified spinal meningiomas: correlation with pathological findings. Skeletal Radiol. 2010;39(4):345–52.

Chapter 18
Surgical Treatment of Epilepsy

Todd S. Trask and Videndra Desai

Epilepsy is broadly defined as recurrent (two or more), unprovoked seizures [1, 2]. More specifically, epilepsy is a disorder characterized by a predisposition to epileptic seizures and by the neurobiologic, cognitive, psychological and social consequences of this disorder [2]. Epilepsy is the most common serious neurological condition, affecting over 60 million people worldwide [3]. Causes of epilepsy are considered multi-factorial, including genetic, acquired influence and provoking factors [4]. Shorvon et al. classifies causes of epilepsy into the following four groups and subgroups [4]:

1. Idiopathic

    (a) Single gene disorders
    (b) Complex inheritance

T.S. Trask, MD (✉)
Department of Neurosurgery,
Methodist Neurological Institute,
6560 Fannin St, Suite 944, Houston, TX 77030, USA
e-mail: ttrask@tmhs.org

V. Desai, MD
Department of Neurosurgery,
Houston Methodist Hospital,
6565 Fannin, Houston, TX 77030, USA

A. Agrawal, G. Britz (eds.), *Emergency Approaches to Neurosurgical Conditions*, DOI 10.1007/978-3-319-10693-9_18,
© Springer International Publishing Switzerland 2015

2. Symptomatic

   (a) Genetic or developmental conditions

        (i)   Childhood epilepsy syndromes
        (ii) Progressive myoclonic epilepsies
        (iii) Neurocutaneous syndromes
        (iv) Single gene or chromosomal disorders
        (v)   Developmental cerebral structural anomalies

   (b) Acquired conditions

        (i)   Hippocampal sclerosis
        (ii) Trauma
        (iii) Tumor
        (iv) Infection
        (v)   Vascular insult
        (vi) Immunological disorders
        (vii) Psychiatric disorders or dementias

3. Provoked

   (a) Provoking factors

        (i)   Fever
        (ii) Menstrual disorders
        (iii) Metabolic or endocrine disturbances

   (b) Reflex epilepsies

        (i)   Photosensitive epilepsy
        (ii) Startle-induced epilepsy
        (iii) Reading/auditory/eating or hot water-induced
              epilepsies

4. Cryptogenic, i.e. unknown causes

The consequences of epilepsy include seizures, cognitive deficits, psychological issues and social/economic issues. Epilepsy patients have poorer self-esteem and higher levels of anxiety and depression, lower rates of marriage and greater rates of social isolation [5]. Some, but not all, epilepsy patients feel stigmatized by their condition [5]. Additionally, epilepsy patients have lower employment rates (one half), higher rates of welfare payments and of those that are employed, incomes are lower relative to people without epilepsy (one half) [5, 6]. Hospital and medication costs are more than double for epileptic patients than non-epileptic patients [6]. They also have a reduced quality of life [6].

There are many antiepileptic medications, and for nearly 80 % of patients, seizures can be controlled with one medication [1]. If treatment with a single medication fails, only about 10 % will benefit from taking multiple medications simultaneously [1]. There are also many side effects of these medications, including drowsiness, confusion, diplopia, liver failure, anemia, thrombocytopenia and more [1].

When medications don't work, which occurs in 1/3 of patients, or when they are associated with too many side effects, surgery may be indicated [7]. The benefit of surgery could be freedom from seizures, but it incurs the risk of losing language function or memory impairment. When choosing patients surgery, the following two criteria are required [7]:

1. Seizures are medically refractory
2. Electrophysiologic, neurologic, neuropsychological and imaging data are concordant with a specific site of seizure origin

    (a) Must demonstrate localization of this site in three or more seizures
    (b) Resection of the site must not cause unacceptable neuro deficit

        (i) Can prognosticate the speech/memory deficit a patient will have with intracarotid amobarbital (Amytal) testing (Wada test)
        (ii) Thus patients who have seizures arising from eloquent cortex, or are multifocal, bilateral or generalized, are not candidates for surgical resection [8].

Planning surgical resection requires many different diagnostic modalities. It includes structural testing, such as MRI, and functional testing, such as the Wada test, functional MRI and electroencephalography (EEG). Structural testing includes MRI, which can be used to depict macroscopic structural abnormalities that can be the source of seizures. It allows the clinician to identify the location of the lesion relative to surrounding structures, which aids the planning of surgical resection. The Wada test, also known as the intra-carotid sodium amobarbital procedure (ISAP), is named after Juhn Atsushi Wada, a Japanese Canadian neurologist who first used it to anesthetize a hemisphere to decrease cognitive side effects associated with bilateral electro-convulsive therapy (ECT). IASP is one of oldest procedures used to prognosticate memory function after temporal lobe resection. IASP results relate to verbal memory changes after surgery but not visuospatial memory changes [9]. IASP is used to assess language dominance and memory competence of each hemisphere in a surgical candidate [10]. The drawbacks of IASP include being invasive, with complications reaching 3 %, as well as only being able to measure the relative distribution of language across two hemispheres (meaning, it only tells how much of language is dominated by one hemisphere relative to other one, not exactly where the language function occurs) [11]. More specific information about localization within one hemisphere must be obtained by intraoperative cortical mapping [11]. It also depends on relatively symmetric and separate arterial supplies for each hemisphere [11].

Because of the drawbacks of IASP, fMRI is steadily replacing it. fMRI has been shown to have good correlation with Wada in lateralizing language function and is non-invasive, has no significant health risks, is not affected by underlying arterial patterns, can be easily repeated without additional risk, affords the examiner sufficient time to test a range of cortical functions and also provides detailed information about spatial localization of functions within each hemisphere [11]. Its limitations include the inability to perform the study in patients with claustrophobia, pacemakers, or those unable to hold still (cognitive or attentional deficits, which may be common in epilepsy patients) [11].

An EEG is also non-invasive, is usually first step in seizure localization, and stratifies patients into the following four groups [7]:

1. Origin of seizure can be lateralized to right or left anterior temporal lobe
2. Bilateral localization
3. Posterior temporal or extra-temporal
4. Unable to localize

Group I patients are candidates for anterior temporal lobectomy while group four patients are candidates for invasive EEG [7]. Invasive EEG involves strip electrodes that are placed through small holes in the temporal bone of the skull into a space just beneath the skull called the subdural space. These electrodes are disc electrodes embedded in silastic (see image below) [7].

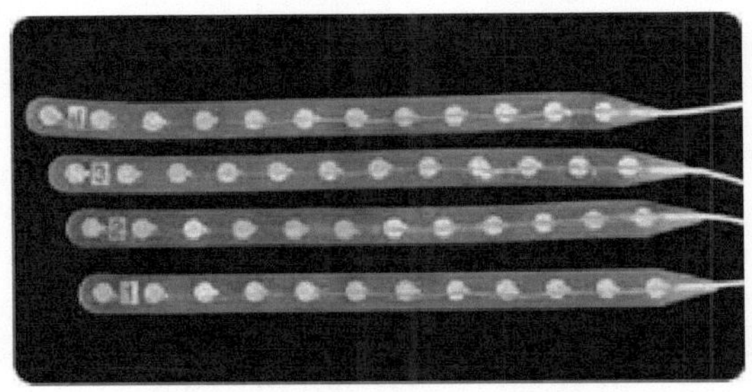

Fluoroscopy is used to confirm adequate placement. The surgeon can also place foramen ovale electrodes through the skin into the "foramen ovale" – a hole at the base of the skull, penetrating dura mater (the tough covering of the cerebral nervous system) and lying adjacent to the mesial temporal lobe (a common site of epileptogenesis) [7]. Subdural strip electrodes are left in place for 4–7 days for seizure recording, depending on surgeon preference, and can be removed under deep conscious sedation with gentle/constant traction (no surgery required) [7].

Depth electrodes are tubular, rigid or semi-rigid electrodes that penetrate brain tissue and are inserted stereotactically into the hippocampus (see image below).

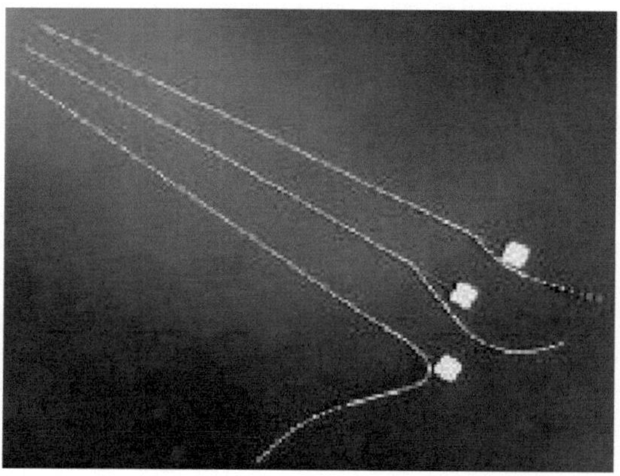

These electrodes are placed with frameless or framed MRI stereotaxy using a route through the back of the head near the midline, in medical jargon an occipital, parasagittal route, so that one electrode can be placed to simultaneously record from both the amygdala and the anterior and posterior parts of the hippocampus [7]. Multimodality imaging of anatomic and angiographic studies can be combined to allow planning of trajectories to avoid vessels and improve safety of placement [7]. For instance, depth electrodes can also be placed orthogonally using an approach through the temporal bone. But blood vessels off the middle cerebral artery can travel inferiorly in the temporal lobe and be at risk of injury with this approach, so many use stereotactic angiography or magnetic resonance angiography or magnetic resonance venography (MRA/MRV). Depth electrodes can also be placed straight down, vertically with a coronal approach, but this is uncommonly used because it requires traversing the internal capsule, the nerve fibers controlling muscular function, to reach the hippocampus. Both subdural and depth electrode types are MRI-compatible [7].

In addition to defining the epileptogenic zone, the surgeon must identify functional cortex, which can be done by mapping the cortex under a grid electrode. Two electrodes in the grid are selected and stimulated with enough current to produce an effect but not so much that there are after-discharges (amount of current varies between different patients and different cortical regions) [7]. If the ictal onset zone (area where seizures initiate) is close to a crucial functional area such as motor speech, one can do an operation with the patient awake in order to map language function and to better identify the boundaries of these two (extra-operative cortical mapping is limited to an accuracy of 1 cm, which is the space between two electrodes) [7].

The most common complication of electrodes is infection –0.85 % if antibiotics are given just prior to surgery. Morbidity is highest with intracranial grids and lowest with strips. Other complications of strip electrodes include cortical contusion, cerebral edema, brain abscess, subdural empyema and subdural hematoma, placement of electrodes into brain parenchyma, accidental extraction of electrodes, superficial wound infection, and permanent neurologic deficit in <1 % [7]. Complications of grid placement are infection, transient neurologic deficit, hematoma, cerebral edema with increased intracranial pressure, and infarction. Transient neurologic deficits occur secondary to edema, hematoma or mass effect from grid, in which case the grid is removed immediately. Complications of depth electrodes are intraparenchymal hemorrhage, subarachnoid hemorrhage, vasospasm and misplacement of the electrode. The electrode can hit the brain stem or posterior cerebral artery, which can be avoided by targeting tip placement in the lateral amygdala and lateral hippocampus, making sure the hole through the occipital bone is not too close to the midline, and confirming the trajectory with an image guidance system before placing the electrode. Alternatively, the electrode can be placed in the temporal horn of the lateral ventricle (adjacent to the hippocampus) with the tip in the amygdala. The risk of permanent neurologic deficit with an occipital approach is <1 % [7].

There are many options for surgical treatment including neuroablation, neuromodulation, and surgical resection. Neuroablation can be performed via radiofrequency thermocoagulation, magnetic resonance-guided focused ultrasound surgery, laser ablation and stereotactic radiosurgery. In radiofrequency (RF) thermocoagulation, a radiofrequency generator is attached to depth electrodes that are placed deep within the brain to the presumed site of epileptogenesis. The generator creates heat by generating a current and thus induces cell death via thermocoagulation. Results are modest with only about 50 % benefiting from surgery, but this may be considered a first-line option for minimally invasive treatment [12]. Magnetic resonance-guided focused ultrasound surgery uses MRI to localize the area of interest, and then ultrasound energy is used to cause a lesion to it. Its strengths include no radiation, currently being non-invasive as no surgery is necessary (previously an opening in the skull was necessary to reduce "defocusing" caused by the skull), no trajectory restrictions and nearly real-time feedback on the lesioning effect via MR thermometry. The main drawback is inadvertent heating of the skull base resulting in injury to cranial nerves [12]. Laser ablation involves MRI-guided laser therapy that uses stereotaxy to guide thermal ablation via a laser. Advantages are that it is more precise than RF thermocoagulation, provides reliable real-time feedback and avoids skull base heating seen in ultrasound energy. The only drawback is that it is invasive, and thus incurs standard surgical risks of infection, hemorrhage, etc. [12]. Stereotactic radiosurgery focuses ionizing radiation to deep lesions with the advantage of being non-invasive but having the drawbacks of radiation (collateral tissue injury and increased risk of future malignancy) and a latent period of efficacy [12].

Within the realm of neuromodulation there is vagal nerve stimulation and deep brain stimulation. Left-sided vagal nerve stimulation (VNS) has been approved for treatment of medically refractory epilepsy as well as treatment-resistant depression, while right-sided VNS has been effective in treating heart failure. The vagus nerve is a mixed cranial nerve that is about 20 % "efferent" (in that it sends signals from the brain to the body) and 80 % "afferent" (relaying information from the body to the brain) [13]. The vagus nerve travels from the brainstem through the neck and chest and into the abdominal cavity, innervating various structures along its route. "Vagus nerve stimulation" describes any technique used to stimulate the vagus nerve – it was first discovered in the 1880s that manual massage/compression of the carotid artery in the neck could suppress seizures, theoretically by stimulating the vagus nerve. Then in the 1930s and 1940s, electrical stimulation of the vagus nerve was shown to affect brain electrical activity in cats and monkeys, and subsequent studies showed anticonvulsant effects on experimentally-induced seizures in dogs. In 1997, the FDA approved surgical implantation of a device to electrically stimulate the vagus nerve for treatment of epilepsy [13].

VNS surgery involves general anesthesia and a programmable pulse generator is implanted in the subcutaneous tissue of the left chest typically. An electrical lead wire is attached to the left vagus nerve in the neck through a second incision. The wire is then tunneled underneath the skin and attached to the generator, and both incisions are sutured closed. Complications include infection and hoarseness due to temporary or permanent left vocal cord paralysis [13]. A small handheld computer is used to program the generator by placing it on the patient's skin over the device and setting certain parameters such as current charge (electrical stimulus intensity measured in milliamperes, mA), pulse width (electrical pulse duration, measured in microseconds), pulse frequency (measured in Hertz, Hz), and the on/off duty cycle (the stimulus on-time and off-time, measured in seconds or minutes). Typically the generator runs continuously, but it can be turned off temporarily by the patient by holding a magnet over the device. It can also be turned on or off by the programmer. The battery life depends on the usage parameters and typically needs replacement every few years via a simple surgical procedure. Side effects of VNS include voice alteration, cough, dyspnea, dysphagia, and neck pain or paresthesia.

Stimulation of only the left vagus nerve is performed because it theoretically reduces effects on the heart such as bradycardia or asystole, since the heart is mainly innervated by the right vagus nerve. These side effects can be minimized by adjusting the parameters of the generator, but tolerance usually occurs via chronic stimulation. Metal detectors, cell phones, microwave ovens and other electronic devices do not affect the generator [13].

Deep brain stimulation involves electrodes placed in different, deep locations within the brain, and they theoretically work by interrupting the propagation of seizures or by increasing overall seizure threshold. Deep brain stimulation (DBS) has also been used for surgical treatment of movement-related disorders such as essential tremor and Parkinson's disease with remarkable success, propelling investigators to apply DBS to epilepsy treatment [14]. Multiple different targets for treating epilepsy with DBS have been studied, including the cerebellum, caudate nucleus, centromedian thalamus, anterior thalamus, subthalamic nucleus and the hippocampus, but only stimulation of the anterior thalamus has thus far received class I evidence for efficacy [14]. Results are modest and stimulation-related side effects such as depression and other psychiatric issues can occur [12].

Epilepsy surgery includes temporal lobectomy, hemispherectomy, and corpus callosotomy. In a temporal lobectomy, the patient is placed in three-point fixation with a Mayfield head holder and fixed to the table with head slightly extended and turned to the side. The scalp is then shaved and cleaned. The incision is made in a question-mark form starting just anterior to the ear, curving over the top of the ear posteriorly and then curving back anteriorly, and stopping just behind the hairline. The scalp is flapped down as well as the temporalis muscle and a large craniotomy is made with the drill. After this, the covering around the brain, the dura mater, is opened and the temporal lobe is identified. Using the microscope, the anterior temporal lobe is resected as planned pre-operatively. One must be cognizant of the structures medial to the temporal lobe including the brain stem, internal carotid artery and several of its important branches, and the third and fourth cranial nerves. Once the resection is complete, hemostasis is achieved and closure is performed [15].

Hemispherectomy was first developed in late 1920s and early 1930s for treatment of large tumors confined to a single hemisphere, but because of the surgical morbidity, it was abandoned. However, it was revived and applied to epilepsy in 1938 till 1960, when again it was less favored secondary to a report showing that after this procedure, superficial coating of the cortex with iron deposits led to mortality. Hemispherectomy should only be performed when the seizures are limited to one hemisphere and multifocal resections in one hemisphere would not be effective [16]. It provides good seizure control (80–90 %) with the risk of iron deposits along the superficial cortex. Because of this, "functional" hemispherectomies began to grow favor [16].

When "eloquent" brain (in other words, tissue with significant function such as motor control or speech function) is involved, resection of the tissue would be disabling. In these cases, or when seizures are caused by multiple bilateral foci, "corpus callosotomy" can be performed. In this procedure, the fibers connecting the two cerebral hemispheres are cut. This procedure is also effective for "drop attacks", where loss of postural tone leads to falling and injury [1].

In summary, epilepsy is a common disorder with many different treatment modalities. Choosing the correct surgical treatment modality involves a careful examination of each case and a multitude of diagnostic tests. Nevertheless, the outcomes after epilepsy surgery have been strong, and we hope that they continue to improve.

References

1. Greenberg MS. Handbook of neurosurgery. 7th ed. Thieme; 2010. Print.
2. Fisher RS, Boas WVE, Blume W, Elger C, Genton P, Lee P, Engel Jr J. Epileptic seizures and epilepsy: definitions proposed by the International League Against Epilepsy (ILAE) and the International Bureau for Epilepsy (IBE). Epilepsia. 2005;46(4):470–2.

 3. Neligan A, Sander JW. Epidemiology of seizures and epilepsy. In: Miller JW, Goodkin HP, editors, Epilepsy. 2013. Print.
 4. Shorvon SD, Andermann F, Guerrini R. The causes of epilepsy: common and uncommon causes in adults and children.
 5. Baker GA, Jacoby A, Buck D, Stalgis C, Monnet D. Quality of life of people with epilepsy: a European study. Epilepsia. 1997;38(3):353–62.
 6. Jennum P, Gyllenborg J, Kjellberg J. The social and economic consequences of epilepsy: a controlled national study. Epilepsia. 2011;52(5):949–56.
 7. Schmidek HH, Roberts DW. Operative neurosurgical techniques: indications, methods and results. 5th ed. Saunders Elsevier; 2006.
 8. Kahane P, Depaulis A. Deep brain stimulation in epilepsy: what is next? Curr Opin Neurol. 2010;23:177–82.
 9. Chiaravalloti ND, Glosser G. Material-specific memory changes after anterior temporal lobectomy as predicted by the intracarotid amobarbital test. Epilepsia. 2001;42(7):902–11.
10. O'Brien TJ, et al. Temporal lobe epilepsy caused by mesial temporal sclerosis and temporal neocortical lesions: a clinical and electroencephalographic study of 46 pathologically proven cases. Brain. 1996;119:2133–41.
11. Binder JR, et al. Determination of language dominance using functional MRI: a comparison with the Wada test. Neurology. 1996;46:978–84.
12. Nowell M, Miserocchi A, McEvoy AW, Duncan JS. Advances in epilepsy surgery. J Neurol Neurosurg Psychiatry. 2014;0:1–7.
13. Howland RH. Vagus nerve stimulation. Curr Behav Neurosci Rep. 2014;1:64–73.
14. Chen XL, Xiong YY, Xu GL, Liu XF. Deep brain stimulation. Intervent Neurol. 2012;1(3–4):200–12.
15. Bejjani GK. Surgical treatment for intractable epilepsy: chapter 68. Atlas of neurosurgical techniques, brain. Thieme; 2006 print.
16. Beier AD, Rutka JT. Hemispherectomy: historical review and recent technical advances. J Neurosurg. 2013;34(6):E11. doi:10.3171/2013.3.FOCUS1341.

Index

A. Agrawal, G. Britz (eds.), *Emergency Approaches to
Neurosurgical Conditions*, DOI 10.1007/978-3-319-10693-9,
© Springer International Publishing Switzerland 2015

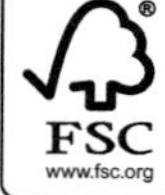

MIX
Papier aus verantwortungsvollen Quellen
Paper from responsible sources
FSC® C105338

If you have any concerns about our products,
you can contact us on
ProductSafety@springernature.com

In case Publisher is established outside the EU,
the EU authorized representative is:
Springer Nature Customer Service Center GmbH
Europaplatz 3, 69115 Heidelberg, Germany

Printed by Libri Plureos GmbH
in Hamburg, Germany